Vital Dyes in Vitreoretinal Surgery

Developments in Ophthalmology

Vol. 42

Series Editor

W. Behrens-Baumann Magdeburg

Vital Dyes in Vitreoretinal Surgery

Chromovitrectomy

Volume Editor

Carsten H. Meyer Bonn

69 figures, 47 in color, and 11 tables, 2008

KARGER

Basel · Freiburg · Paris · London · New York · Bangalore · Bangkok · Shanghai · Singapore · Tokyo · Sydney

Carsten H. Meyer

Department of Ophthalmology
University of Bonn
Ernst-Abbe-Strasse 2
DE–53127 Bonn

Library of Congress Cataloging-in-Publication Data

Vital dyes in vitreoretinal surgery : chromovitrectomy/volume editor,
Carsten H. Meyer
p. ; cm. – (Developments in ophthalmology, ISSN 0250-3751 ; v. 42)
Includes bibliographical references and indexes.
ISBN 978-3-8055-8551-4 (hard cover : alk. paper)
1. Vitreous body–Surgery. 2. Vitrectomy. 3. Retina–Diseases. 4. Dyes
and dyeing–Therapeutic use. I. Meyer, Carsten H. II. Title:
Chromovitrectomy. III. Series.
[DNLM: 1. Vitreous Body–Surgery. 2. Coloring Agents–therapeutic use.
3. Retina–surgery. 4. Vitrectomy–methods. W1 DE998NG v. 42 2008 / ww 250
v836 2008]
RE501. v56 2008
617.7'46–dc22

2008014732

Bibliographic Indices. This publication is listed in bibliographic services, including Current Contents®

Drug Dosage. The authors and the publisher have exerted every effort to ensure that drug selection and dosage set forth in this text are in accord with current recommendations and practice at the time of publication. However, in view of ongoing research, changes in government regulations, and the constant flow of information relating to drug therapy and drug reactions, the reader is urged to check the package insert for each drug for any change in indications and dosage and for added warnings and precautions. This is particularly important when the recommended agent is a new and/or infrequently employed drug.

www.karger.com
Printed in Switzerland on acid-free and non-aging paper (ISO 9706) by Reinhardt Druck, Basel
ISSN 0250–3751
ISBN: 978–3–8055–8551–4

Contents

VII List of Contributors

XI Preface
Meyer, C.H. (Bonn)

1 A Vitrectomy Is Done, When the Vitreous Is Gone! A Tribute to Prof. Peter Kroll
Meyer, C.H. (Bonn)

5 To See the Invisible: The Quest of Imaging Vitreous
Sebag, J. (Los Angeles, Calif.)

29 Historical Aspects and Evolution of the Application of Vital Dyes in Vitreoretinal Surgery and Chromovitrectomy
Rodrigues, E.B.; Penha, F.M.; Furlani, B. (Sao Paulo); Meyer, C.H. (Bonn); Maia, M.; Farah, M.E. (Sao Paulo)

35 Three Simple Approaches to Visualize the Transparent Vitreous Cortex during Vitreoretinal Surgery
Schmidt, J.C.; Chofflet, J.; Hörle, S.; Mennel, S.; Meyer, C.H. (Marburg)

43 Safety Parameters for Indocyanine Green in Vitreoretinal Surgery
Grisanti, S. (Tübingen, Luebeck); Altvater, A. (Tübingen); Peters, S. (Tübingen, Luebeck)

69 Toxicity of Indocyanine Green in Vitreoretinal Surgery
Gandorfer, A.; Haritoglou, C.; Kampik, A. (Munich)

82 Biomechanical Changes of the Internal Limiting Membrane after Indocyanine Green Staining
Wollensak, G. (Berlin)

91 Current Concepts of Trypan Blue in Chromovitrectomy
Farah, M.E.; Maia, M.; Furlani, B.; Bottós, J.; Meyer, C.H.; Lima, V.; Penha, F.M.; Costa, E.F.; Rodrigues, E.B. (Sao Paulo)

101 **Trityl Dyes Patent Blue V and Brilliant Blue G – Clinical Relevance and in vitro Analysis of the Function of the Outer Blood-Retinal Barrier**
Mennel, S. (Marburg); Meyer, C.H. (Bonn); Schmidt, J.C. (Marburg); Kaempf, S.; Thumann, G. (Aachen)

115 **Brilliant Blue in Vitreoretinal Surgery**
Enaida, H.; Ishibashi, T. (Fukuoka)

126 **Vital Staining and Retinal Detachment Surgery**
Jackson, T.L. (London)

141 **An Experimental Approach towards Novel Dyes for Intraocular Surgery**
Haritoglou, C.; Schüttauf, F.; Gandorfer, A.; Thaler, S. (Munich/Tübingen)

153 **Experimental Evaluation of Microplasmin – An Alternative to Vital Dyes**
Gandorfer, A. (Munich)

160 **Author Index**

161 **Subject Index**

List of Contributors

Andreas Altvater
University Eye Hospital
Center for Ophthalmology
Eberhard-Karls-University of Tübingen
Schleichstrasse 12–15
DE–72076 Tübingen (Germany)

Juliana Bottós
Federal University of Sao Paulo
Vision Institute
Department of Ophthalmology
Sao Paulo (Brazil)

Jack Chofflet
92, Chemin St. Christophe
FR-06130 Grasse (France)

Elaine F. Costa
Federal University of Sao Paulo
Vision Institute,
Department of Ophthalmology
Sao Paulo (Brazil)

Hirsoshi Enaida
Department of Ophthalmology
Clinical Research Institute
National Hospital Organization
Kyushu Medical Center
1-8-1 Jigyohama, Chuo-ku
Fukuoka, 801-8563 (Japan)

Michel E. Farah
Federal University of Sao Paulo
Vision Institute
Department of Ophthalmology
Sao Paulo (Brazil)

Bruno Furlani
Federal University of Sao Paulo
Vision Institute
Department of Ophthalmology
Sao Paulo (Brazil)

Arnd Gandorfer
Department of Ophthalmology
Ludwig-Maximilians-University
Mathildenstrasse 8
DE–80336 Munich (Germany)

Salvatore Grisanti
Department of Ophthalmology
Universitätsklinikum Schleswig-Holstein
Campus Luebeck
Ratzeburger Allee 160
DE–23538 Luebeck (Germany)

Christos Haritoglou
Department of Ophthalmology
Ludwig-Maximilians-University
Mathildenstrasse 8
DE–80336 Munich (Germany)

Steffen Hörle
Department of Ophthalmology
Philipps-University Marburg
Robert-Koch-Strasse 4
DE–35037 Marburg (Germany)

Tatsuro Ishibashi, MD
Department of Ophthalmology
Graduate School of Medical Sciences
Kyushu University
3–1–1 Maidashi, Higashi-ku
Fukuoka, 812–8582 (Japan)

Timothy L. Jackson
Department of Ophthalmology
King's College Hospital
London SE5 9RS (UK)

Stefanie Kaempf
IZKF 'Biomat'
Department of Ophthalmology
Rheinisch-Westfälische Technische
Hochschule Aachen
Pauwelsstrasse 30
52074 Aachen (Germany)

Anselm Kampik
Department of Ophthalmology
Ludwig-Maximilians-University
Mathildenstrasse 8
DE–80336 Munich (Germany)

Veronica Lima
Federal University of Sao Paulo
Vision Institute
Department of Ophthalmology
Sao Paulo (Brazil)

Mauricio Maia
Federal University of Sao Paulo
Vision Institute
Department of Ophthalmology
Sao Paulo (Brazil)

Stefan Mennel
Department of Ophthalmology
Philipps-University Marburg
Robert-Koch-Strasse 4
DE–35037 Marburg (Germany)

Carsten H. Meyer
Department of Ophthalmology
University of Bonn
Ernst-Abbe-Strasse 2
DE–53127 Bonn (Germany)

Fernando M. Penha
Federal University of Sao Paulo
Vision Institute
Department of Ophthalmology
Sao Paulo (Brazil)

Swaantje Peters
Department of Ophthalmology
Universitätsklinikum Schleswig-Holstein
Campus Luebeck
Ratzeburger Allee 160
DE–23538 Luebeck (Germany)

Eduardo B. Rodrigues, MD
Rua Presidente Coutinho 579
conj 501
Florianópolis
SC 88015–300 (Brazil)

Jörg C. Schmidt
Department of Ophthalmology
Philipps-University Marburg
Robert-Koch-Strasse 4
DE–35037 Marburg (Germany)

Frank Schüttauf
University Eye Hospital
Center for Ophthalmology
Eberhard-Karls-University of Tübingen
Schleichstrasse 12–15
DE–72076 Tübingen (Germany)

Jerry Sebag
VMR Institute
University of Southern California
7677 Center Avenue
Huntington Beach, CA 92647 (USA)

Sebastian Thaler
University Eye Hospital
Center for Ophthalmology
Eberhard-Karls-University of Tübingen
Schleichstrasse 12–15
DE–72076 Tübingen (Germany)

Gabi Thumann
Department of Ophthalmology
Rheinisch-Westfälische Technische
Hochschule Aachen
Pauwelsstrasse 30
52074 Aachen (Germany)

Gregor Wollensak
Wildentensteig 4
DE–14195 Berlin (Germany)

Preface

Indocyanine green (ICG) has a high affinity to the internal limiting membrane (ILM) of the retina. However, its potential toxicity to the retina and unclear side effects opened a wide discussion on the benefit and complications of any vital dye in vitreoretinal surgery (chromovitrectomy). This book highlights the major clinical and experimental results with currently used novel vital dyes in modern vitreoretinal surgery. The first three chapters describe the transparent structure of the vitreous body and summarize historical considerations to visualize its structure by optical coherence tomography, dye injections or autologous cells during surgery for diagnostic purposes. The following three chapters describe the advantages and disadvantages of ICG during vitreoretinal surgery and experimental applications. Alternative approaches by recently approved vital dyes such as trypan blue, patent blue and brilliant blue are evaluated in the subsequent three chapters. The last three chapters give an outlook on novel vital dyes, which are currently under evaluation, as well as alternative enzymatic approaches to remove the vitreous from the retinal surface.

Chromovitrectomy is a novel approach to visualize the vitreous or retinal surface during vitreoretinal surgery. Numerous vital dyes have been applied in experimental settings with promising or devastating results. The widely used ICG has made the surgical maneuver of ILM peeling tremendously safer and efficient. However, its 'off-label' application and ongoing reports on possible side effects make the search for a safer approach necessary. Several alternative vital dyes have already been approved by the industry for vitreoretinal application, while additional dyes are still under evaluation. The authors would like to thank the international research community, governmental funding and private organizations as well as our industrial partners, who have supported this ongoing research over the past decade. The future will show which dye allows the safest approach with possibly no side effects, a high specific affinity for the ILM or other vitreoretinal tissues and the best visual outcome for our patients.

The authors would like to thank the international research community, governmental funding and private organizations as well as our industrial partners (Geuder, Fluoron, Acritec/Zeiss) who have supported this ongoing research over the past decade.

Prof. Dr. med. Carsten H. Meyer,
Bonn

Meyer CH (ed): Vital Dyes in Vitreoretinal Surgery.
Dev Ophthalmol. Basel, Karger, 2008, vol 42, pp 1–4

A Vitrectomy Is Done, When the Vitreous Is Gone!

A Tribute to Prof. Peter Kroll

Carsten H. Meyer

Department of Ophthalmology, University of Bonn, Bonn, Germany

It is my personal pleasure to congratulate Prof. Peter Kroll, a leader in vitreoretinal surgery, on his 65th birthday. Prof. Kroll completed his residency in Ophthalmology at the University of Bonn, Germany, in 1978 and later joined the faculty at the University Eye Clinic in Münster, Germany, where in 1983 he obtained his professorship.

Vitreoretinal surgery was a young subspecialty in ocular surgery at that time with only a first generation of surgical instruments and a limited number of performing vitreoretinal surgeons worldwide. Rotterdam was then a leading center in Europe under the head of Prof. Reljy Zivojnovic, thus Peter Kroll as a young vitreoretinal physician took the initiative to travel from Münster to Rotterdam each week, to see and learn as much as he could from this pioneer in vitreoretinal surgery. His teacher Zivojnovic, known for his success in severe cases of diabetic retinopathy, retinal detachment and ocular trauma, taught him to remove as much vitreous as possible during the vitrectomy and Peter Kroll kept Zivojnovic's secret in mind: *'a vitrectomy is done, when the vitreous is gone.'*

In 1989, Prof. Peter Kroll became the chairman of the Department of Ophthalmology at the Philipps-Universität in Marburg, Germany. He implemented substantial innovations in modern vitreoretinal surgery and made his own remarkable contributions toward the understanding and treatment of diabetic retinopathy [1–3]. His pioneering classification of proliferative diabetic vitreoretinopathy played a critical role in understanding of the vitreous in the pathogenesis of diabetic retinopathy and led to better outcomes after early vitrectomy in rapidly progressing diabetic vitreoretinopathy [4, 5]. His clinical observations were underlined by well-known histological examinations from Faulborn and Duncker [6] as well as his close friend Jerry Sebag [7, 8], who demonstrated the cleavage plane between the vitreoretinal interface and the retinal surface, highlighting the key influence for the vitreoretinal interface in proliferative diabetic vitreoretinopathy.

In the past decade, Prof. Kroll has perfected the concept of a complete vitreous removal by an early vitrectomy with numerous innovations [9–11]. A new generation of better and smaller vitreoretinal instruments has helped him to reduce the ocular trauma during vitreoretinal surgery. Inspiring discussions between close buddies Peter Kroll and Jerry Sebag highlighted the role of vitreopapillary traction [12–14], the spontaneous release of epiretinal membrane [15] as well as the enzymatical release of vitreous traction in diabetic retinopathy [16, 17]. Both were among the pioneers of pharmacological vitrectomy in the mid 1990s. Kroll and Hesse injected recombinant tissue plasminogen activator into the midvitreous to induce a posterior vitreous detachment prior to vitrectomy in diabetic vitreoretinopathy [18–20], while Sebag preferred other enzymes, for example plasmin and later microplasmin, to induce a posterior vitreous detachment [21].

In 1998, Burk et al. [22] proposed the injection of indocyanine green into the vitreous cavity in order to stain the inner limiting membrane during vitrectomy. This procedure allows a better visualization and complete removal of the inner limiting membrane, and is currently used by most surgeons. However, when numerous authors described a variety of possible adverse events [23–25], a new search for alternative dyes began. For a long time, there had been no term to describe the staining of vitreoretinal tissue during vitrectomy, although indocyanine green, trypan blue and patent blue were frequently used. A search in the internet showed us that gastrologists had for more than 20 years used a variety of vital dyes in endoscopy, calling this procedure 'chromoendoscopy'. Thus, Prof. Kroll proposed with his pioneer talk 'The magic colors in chromovitrectomy' at the Vail meeting 2002 to generally call the application of any vital dyes during vitrectomy 'chromovitrectomy' [26].

Throughout more than two decades, Prof. Kroll had attracted patients and colleagues from all over the world and gathered a group of young talented vitreoretinal physicians to perform outstanding vitreoretinal surgery in Marburg. He is the founder of the vitreoretinal symposium (VRS), which is hosted in Germany each year for well-known vitreoretinal surgeons from around the world. The close formatted discussion between presenter and audience gives this meeting a unique platform to exchange ideas and novel opinions. But even if one does not have the great privilege to talk to him during the VRS, one might have the chance after the lectures at the great evening gala to which Prof. Kroll, being a generous host, invites all speakers and participants of the congress. Many of us have enjoyed celebrating with him at any one of these evening galas.

As a gifted surgeon, physician and teacher, Prof. Kroll made many contributions affecting our daily work. For good reason, his achievements have earned him worldwide recognition. The generation of vitreoretinal specialists he has trained will strive to replicate his unyielding energy, his devotion to surgical training and his unbending sense of morality. He has taught each of us important skill, and enhanced the care of our patients tremendously. He has cared about each of us individually. The creative ideas of Peter Kroll have led to pioneering landmarks in the field of diabetic vitreoretinopathy and modern vitreoretinal surgery. He is a great teacher and he

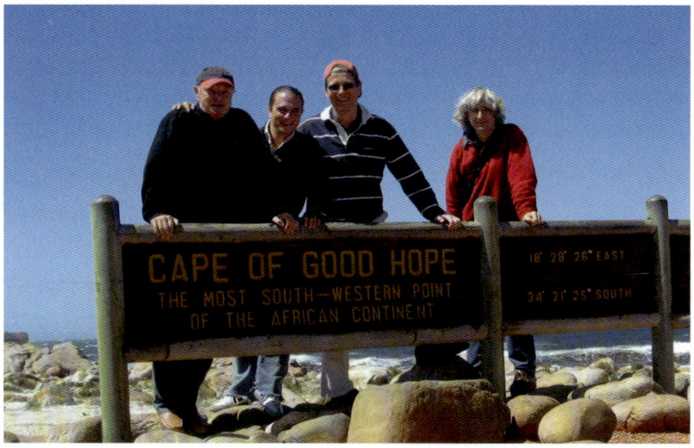
CAPE OF GOOD HOPE
THE MOST SOUTH-WESTERN POINT
OF THE AFRICAN CONTINENT

Fig. 1. Going to the limits: excursion to the Cape of Good Hope during the Meeting of the Club Jules Gonin in Cape Town in 2006. From left to right: Prof. Kroll, his son Dr. Tobias Kroll, Prof. Carsten Meyer and Prof. Jörg Schmidt.

forced his fellows and attendings to go to the limits and search for new frontiers in vitreoretinal surgery. A special time with him was witnessed in South Africa, when he showed us 'Cape of Good Hope', the most southern point of Africa. What a day to remember (fig. 1)! Prof. Kroll obtained important principles about successful vitreoretinal surgery from well-known surgeons such as Reljy Zivojnovic, Boja Corcostegui and Steve Charles. Convinced by the concept of a complete vitrectomy, he developed additional techniques to minimize surgical trauma by injecting enzymes or vital dyes in the vitreous cavity. He transferred his knowledge and long experience to his fellows and attendings who are grateful to him for helping them to achieve a safer approach and better functional outcome for their patients.

With this book, we would like to honor Prof. Kroll's lifetime achievements and thank him for all he has done for us personally and for our careers. He is a compassionate individual and the tributes you will read in this volume will only begin to highlight how much each of us appreciates him. I have always felt that he has been most influential on my career and for that I am grateful. On a personal note, I cannot express strongly enough my personal thanks for his support. *Ad multos annos!* All the best to Peter Kroll.

References

1 Kroll P, Rodrigues EB, Hörle S: Pathogenesis and classification of proliferative diabetic vitreoretinopathy. Ophthalmologica 2007;221:78–94.

2 Hörle S, Kroll P: Evidence-based therapy of diabetic retinopathy. Ophthalmologica 2007;221:132–141.

3 Hesse L, Heller G, Kraushaar N, Wesp A, Schröder B, Kroll P: The predictive value of a classification for proliferative diabetic vitreoretinopathy. Klin Monatsbl Augenheilkd 2002;219:46–49.

4 Hesse L, Bodanowitz S, Huhnermann M, Kroll P: Prediction of visual acuity after early vitrectomy in diabetics. Ger J Ophthalmol 1996;5:257–261.

5 Hörle S, Pöstgens H, Schmidt J, Kroll P: Effect of pars plana vitrectomy for proliferative diabetic vitreoretinopathy on preexisting diabetic maculopathy. Graefes Arch Clin Exp Ophthalmol 2002;240: 197–201.

6 Faulborn J, Dunker S, Bowald S: Diabetic vitreopathy – Findings using the celloidin embedding technique. Ophthalmologica 1998;212:369–376.

7 Sebag J, Ansari RR, Dunker S, Suh KI: Dynamic light scattering of diabetic vitreopathy. Diabetes Technol Ther 1999;1:169–176.

8 Sebag J: Diabetic vitreopathy. Ophthalmology 1996; 103:205–206.

9 Schmidt JC, Nietgen GW, Hesse L, Kroll P: External diaphanoscopic illuminator: a new device for visualization in pars plana vitrectomy. Retina 2000;20: 103–106.

10 Meyer CH, Rodrigues EB, Schmidt JC, Hörle S, Kroll P: Sutureless vitrectomy surgery. Ophthalmology 2003; 110:2427–2428.

11 Schmidt J, Nietgen GW, Brieden S: Self-sealing, sutureless sclerotomy in pars-plana vitrectomy. Klin Monatsbl Augenheilkd 1999;215:247–251.

12 Kroll P, Wiegand W, Schmidt J: Vitreopapillary traction in proliferative diabetic vitreoretinopathy. Br J Ophthalmol 1999;83:261–264.

13 Sebag J: Vitreopapillary traction as a cause of elevated optic nerve head. Am J Ophthalmol 1999;128: 261–262.

14 Meyer CH, Schmidt JC, Mennel S, Kroll P: Functional and anatomical results of vitreopapillary traction after vitrectomy. Acta Ophthalmol Scand 2007; 85:221–222.

15 Meyer CH, Rodrigues EB, Mennel S, Schmidt JC, Kroll P: Spontaneous separation of epiretinal membrane in young subjects: personal observations and review of the literature. Graefes Arch Clin Exp Ophthalmol 2004;242:977–985.

16 Hesse L, Chofflet J, Kroll P: Tissue plasminogen activator as a biochemical adjuvant in vitrectomy for proliferative diabetic vitreoretinopathy. Ger J Ophthalmol 1995;4:323–327.

17 Sebag J: Pharmacologic vitreolysis. Retina 1998;18: 1–3.

18 Hesse L, Kroll P: Enzymatically induced posterior vitreous detachment in proliferative diabetic vitreoretinopathy. Klin Monatsbl Augenheilkd 1999;214: 84–89.

19 Hesse L, Kroll P: TPA-assisted vitrectomy for proliferative diabetic retinopathy. Retina 2000;20:317–318.

20 Hesse L, Nebeling B, Schröder B, Heller G, Kroll P: Induction of posterior vitreous detachment in rabbits by intravitreal injection of tissue plasminogen activator following cryopexy. Exp Eye Res 2000; 70:31–39.

21 Sebag J, Ansari RR, Suh KI: Pharmacologic vitreolysis with microplasmin increases vitreous diffusion coefficients. Graefes Arch Clin Exp Ophthalmol 2007; 245:576–580.

22 Schmidt JC, Meyer CH, Rodrigues EB, Hörle S, Kroll P: Staining of internal limiting membrane in vitreomacular surgery: a simplified technique. Retina 2003;23:263–264.

23 Sebag J: Indocyanine green-assisted macular hole surgery: too pioneering? Am J Ophthalmol 2004;137: 744–746.

24 Mennel S, Thumann G, Peter S, Meyer CH, Kroll P: Influence of vital dyes on the function of the outer blood-retinal barrier in vitro. Klin Monatsbl Augenheilkd 2006;223:568–576.

Prof. Dr. Carsten H. Meyer
Department of Ophthalmology, University of Bonn
Ernst-Abbe-Strasse 2
DE–53127 Bonn (Germany)
E-Mail meyer_eye@yahoo.com

Meyer CH (ed): Vital Dyes in Vitreoretinal Surgery.
Dev Ophthalmol. Basel, Karger, 2008, vol 42, pp 5–28

To See the Invisible: The Quest of Imaging Vitreous

J. Sebag

VMR Institute, University of Southern California, Los Angeles, Calif., USA

Abstract

Purpose: Imaging vitreous has long been a quest to view what is, by design, invisible. This chapter will review important historical aspects, past and present imaging methodologies, and new technologies that are currently in development for future research and clinical applications. **Methods:** Classic and modern histologic techniques, dark-field slit microscopy, clinical slit lamp biomicroscopy, standard and scanning laser ophthalmoscopy (SLO), ultrasonography, optical coherence tomography (OCT), combined OCT-SLO, magnetic resonance and Raman spectroscopies, and dynamic light scattering methodologies are presented. **Results:** The best available histologic techniques for imaging vitreous are those that avoid rapid dehydration of vitreous specimens. Dark-field slit microscopy enables in vitro imaging without dehydration or tissue fixatives. OCT enables better in vivo visualization of the vitreoretinal interface than SLO and ultrasonography, but does not adequately image the vitreous body. The combination of OCT with SLO has provided useful new imaging capabilities, but only at the vitreoretinal interface. Dynamic light scattering can evaluate the vitreous body by determining the average sizes of vitreous macromolecules in aging, disease, and as a means to assess the effects of pharmacologic vitreolysis. Raman spectroscopy can detect altered vitreous molecules, such as glycated collagen and other proteins in diabetic vitreopathy and possibly other diseases. **Conclusions:** A better understanding of normal vitreous physiology and structure and how these change in aging and disease is needed to develop more effective therapies and prevention. The quest to adequately image vitreous will likely only succeed through the combined use of more than one technique to provide better vitreous imaging for future research and clinical applications.

Historical Perspective

Clear by design (fig. 1), vitreous has fascinated men for years. Among the early theories of vitreous structure that were reviewed by Duke-Elder [1] is a description that vitreous is composed of 'loose and delicate filaments surrounded by fluid'. This is remarkably close to present-day concepts. During the 18th and 19th centuries, however, there were no less than four very different theories of vitreous structure. In 1741, Demours formulated the *alveolar theory*, claiming that there are alveoli of fluid

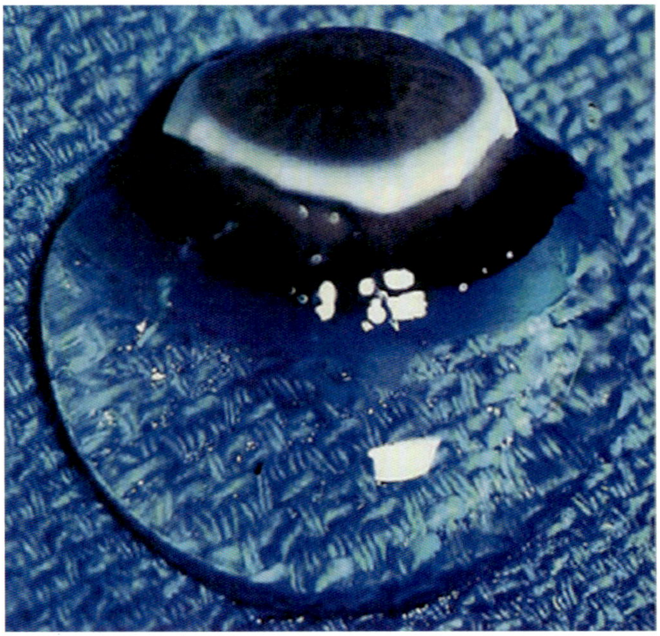

Fig. 1. Human vitreous body of a 9-month-old child dissected of the sclera, choroid, and retina, still attached to the anterior segment. Although the specimen is placed on a surgical towel in room air, the vitreous maintains its shape, because in youth the vitreous body is nearly entirely gel. Specimen courtesy of the New England Eye Bank.

between fibrillar structures. In 1780, Zinn proposed that vitreous is arranged in a concentric, lamellar configuration similar to the layers of an onion. The dissections and histologic preparations of Von Pappenheim and Brucke provided evidence for this *lamellar theory*. The *radial sector theory* was proposed by Hannover in 1845. Studying coronal sections at the equator, he described a multitude of sectors approximately radially oriented around the central anteroposterior core that contains Cloquet's canal. Hannover likened this structure to the appearance of a 'cut orange'. In 1848, Sir William Bowman established the *fibrillar theory*, which was based upon his finding microscopic fibrils, an observation which confirmed Retzius's earlier description of fibers that arose in the peripheral anterior vitreous and assumed an undulating pattern in the central vitreous, similar to a 'horse's tail'. In 1917, the elegant histologic preparations of Szent-Györgi supported these observations and introduced the concept that vitreous structure changes with age.

Unfortunately, the techniques employed in all these studies were flawed by artifacts that biased the results of the investigations. As pointed out by Baurmann and Redslob [2], these early histologic studies employed acid tissue fixatives that precipitated what we recognize today as the glycosaminoglycans hyaluronan (HA; formerly called hyaluronic acid), an effect which altered the histologic imaging of vitreous. Thus, the development of slit lamp biomicroscopy by Gullstrand in 1912 held great promise, as it was anticipated that this technique could enable imaging of vitreous structure without the introduction of fixation artifacts. Yet, as described by Redslob [2], a varied set of descriptions resulted over the years, ranging from a fibrous structure to sheets, 'chain-linked fences', and various other interpretations. This problem even persisted in more recent investigations. Eisner [3] described 'membranelles', Worst [4] 'cisterns', Sebag and Balazs [5] 'fibers', and Kishi and Shimizu [6] 'pockets' in the vitreous. The observation of these so-called 'pockets' by the last-mentioned group was ultimately found to be an age-related phenomenon with little relevance to the normal macromolecular structure [7].

Vitreous Biochemistry

That vitreous is now considered an important ocular structure with respect to both normal physiology [8] as well as several important pathologic conditions of the posterior segment [9] is due in no small part to a better understanding of the biochemical composition and organization of vitreous. Vitreous biochemistry has been extensively reviewed elsewhere [10–12]. The features of vitreous biochemistry that are most relevant to this thesis concern the macromolecules HA and collagen, because these are the major constituents of vitreous along with water.

Hyaluronan

HA is a major macromolecule of vitreous. Although it is present throughout the body, HA was first isolated from bovine vitreous in 1934 by Meyer and Palmer. HA is a long, unbranched polymer of repeating disaccharide (glucuronic acid β-(1,3)-N-acetylglucosamine) moieties linked by β(1–4) bonds [13]. It is a linear, left-handed, threefold helix with a rise per disaccharide on the helix axis of 0.98 nm [14]. The sodium salt of HA has a molecular weight of $3–4.5 \times 10^6$ in normal human vitreous [15]. HA is not normally a free polymer in vivo, but is covalently linked to a protein core, the ensemble being called a proteoglycan.

Collagen

Recent studies [12] of pepsinized forms of collagen confirmed that vitreous contains collagen type II, a hybrid of types V/XI, and type IX collagen in a molar ratio of 75:10:15, respectively. In the entire body, only cartilage has as high a proportion of type II collagen as vitreous, explaining why certain inborn errors of type II collagen metabolism affect vitreous as well as joints. Vitreous collagens are organized into fibrils with type V/XI residing in the core, type II collagen surrounding the core, and type IX collagen on the surface of the fibril. The fibrils are 7–28 nm in diameter [16] but their length in situ is unknown.

Supramolecular Organization

As originally proposed by Balazs and more recently described with precision by Mayne [17], vitreous is a dilute meshwork of collagen fibrils interspersed with extensive arrays of HA molecules. The collagen fibrils provide a scaffold-like structure that is 'inflated' by the hydrophilic HA. If collagen is removed, the remaining HA forms a viscous solution; if HA is removed, the gel shrinks, but is not destroyed. On the basis of this and other observations, Comper and Laurent [18] proposed that electrostatic binding occurs between the negatively charged HA and the positively charged collagen in the vitreous.

Bishop [12] has proposed that to appreciate how vitreous gel is organized and stabilized requires an understanding of what prevents collagen fibrils from aggregating and by what means the collagen fibrils are connected to maintain a stable gel structure. Studies [12] have shown that the chondroitin sulfate chains of type IX collagen bridge between adjacent collagen fibrils in a ladder-like configuration spacing them apart. Such spacing is necessary for vitreous transparency, since keeping vitreous collagen fibrils separated by at least one wavelength of incident light minimizes light scattering, allowing the unhindered transmission of light to the retina for photoreception. Bishop [12] proposed that the leucine-rich repeat protein opticin is the predominant structural protein responsible for short-range spacing of collagen fibrils. Concerning long-range spacing, Scott et al. [19] and Mayne et al. [20] have claimed that HA plays a pivotal role in stabilizing the vitreous gel.

Several types of collagen-HA interactions may occur in different circumstances. Further investigation must be undertaken to identify the nature of collagen-HA interaction in vitreous. This question is important for an understanding of normal vitreous anatomy and physiology, but also as a means by which to understand the biochemical basis for age- and disease-related vitreous liquefaction and posterior vitreous detachment (PVD).

Vitreous Embryology

Interfaces

During invagination of the optic vesicle, the basal lamina of the surface ectoderm enters the invagination along with ectodermal cells that become specialized neural ectoderm. The cells lining the inner surface of the posterior wall of the optic vesicle (the posterior portion of the vesicle that does not invaginate) give rise to retinal pigment epithelium and its basal lamina, Bruch's membrane. The neural ectoderm that accompanies the invaginating anterior wall of the optic vesicle gives rise to the neural retinal cells and their underlying basal lamina, the internal limiting lamina (ILL). Thus, the basal laminae of both the retina and retinal pigment epithelium have the

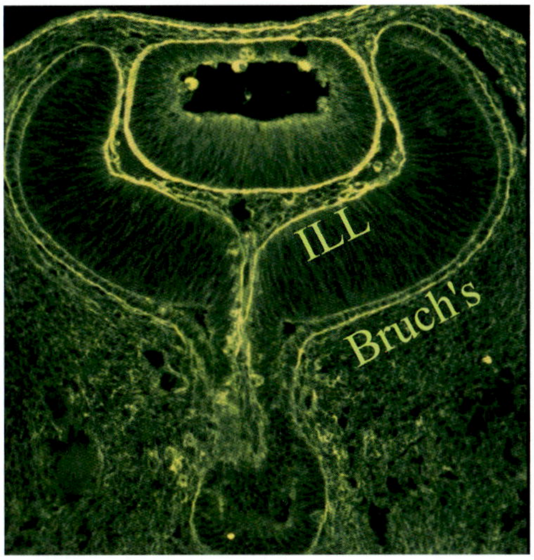

Fig. 2. Embryonic human eye. Posterior to the ILL is the neural retina. The tissue between the lens and the ILL will give rise to the vitreous. Anterior to Bruch's membrane is the retinal pigment epithelium. Of note is the fact that the ILL and Bruch's membrane are continuous, indeed the same structure. The indistinguishable origin of the ILL and Bruch's membrane is important in understanding neovascular (and perhaps other) pathologies of the vitreoretinal interface and the chorioretinal interface.

same embryologic origin. Figure 2 demonstrates the continuity of these two basal laminae. It is important to appreciate that these basal laminae serve as interfaces [21] between adjacent ocular structures. In the case of the ILL, this basal lamina is the interface between the retina and vitreous. Bruch's membrane separates the retinal pigment epithelium and retina from the choroid (neural crest origin).

These interfaces play an important role in a significant biological event that underlies one of the most devastating causes of blindness in humans, i.e. neovascularization. At the ILL interface between vitreous and retina, neovascularization in advanced diabetic retinopathy [22] and other ischemic retinopathies, including retinopathy of prematurity, is a significant cause of vision loss. At the level of Bruch's membrane, an interface of identical embryologic origin as the ILL, neovascularization in age-related macular degeneration is a significant and growing problem. Both of these conditions result from vascular endothelial cell migration and proliferation onto and into interfaces of the same embryologic origin – the basal lamina of the surface ectoderm. Improving our understanding of endothelial cell interaction with these interfaces should provide new insights into therapy and prevention of these important disorders.

Embryology of the Vitreous Body

Early in embryogenesis, the vitreous body is filled with blood vessels known as the vasa hyaloidea propia. This network of vessels arises from the hyaloid artery, which is directly connected to the central retinal artery at the optic disk. The vessels branch many times within the vitreous body and anastomose anteriorly with a network of vessels surrounding the lens, the tunica vasculosa lentis. This embryonic vascular system attains its maximum prominence during the 9th week of gestation or 40-mm stage [23]. Atrophy of the vessels begins posteriorly with dropout of the vasa hyaloidea propria, followed by the tunica vasculosa lentis. At the 240-mm stage (7th month) in human beings, blood flow in the hyaloid artery ceases [24]. Regression of the vessel itself begins with glycogen and lipid deposition in the endothelial cells and pericytes of the hyaloid vessels [24]. Endothelial cell processes then fill the lumen and macrophages form a plug that occludes the vessel. The cells in the vessel wall then undergo necrosis and are phagocytized by mononuclear phagocytes [25]. Gloor [26], however, claimed that macrophages are not involved in vessel regression within the embryonic vitreous but that autolytic vacuoles form in the cells of the vessel walls, perhaps in response to hyperoxia. Interestingly, the sequence of cell disappearance from the primary vitreous begins with endothelial and smooth muscle cells of the vessel walls, followed by adventitial fibroblasts and lastly phagocytes [27], consistent with a gradient of decreasing oxygen tension.

It is not known precisely what stimulates regression of the hyaloid vascular system, but studies have identified a protein native to the vitreous that inhibits angiogenesis in various experimental models [28–31]. Teleologically, such activity seems necessary if a transparent tissue is to inhibit cell migration and proliferation and minimize light scattering to maintain transparency. This may also be the mechanism that induces regression of the vasa hyaloidea propia. Thus, activation of this protein and its effect on the primary vitreous may be responsible for the regression of the embryonic hyaloid vascular system as well as the inhibition of pathologic neovascularization in the adult. Hyaloid vessel regression may also result from a shift in the balance between growth factors promoting new vessels, such as vascular endothelial growth factor A, and those inducing regression, such as placental growth factor.

Recent studies [32, 33] have suggested that the vasa hyaloidea propria and tunica vasculosa lentis regress via apoptosis. Mitchell et al. [32] pointed out that the first event in hyaloid vasculature regression is endothelial cell apoptosis and proposed that lens development separates the fetal vasculature from vascular endothelial growth factor-producing cells, decreasing the levels of this survival factor for vascular endothelium, inducing apoptosis. Following endothelial cell apoptosis, there is loss of capillary integrity, leakage of erythrocytes into the vitreous, and phagocytosis of apoptotic endothelium by macrophages, which were felt to be important in this process. Subsequent studies by a different group [34] confirmed the importance of macrophages in promoting regression of the fetal vitreous vasculature and further characterized these macrophages as hyalocytes. Meeson et al. [35] proposed that there are actually two forms of apoptosis that are important in regression of the fetal vitreous vasculature. The first ('initiating apoptosis') results from macrophage induction of apoptosis in a single endothelial cell of an otherwise healthy capillary segment with normal blood flow. The isolated dying endothelial cells project into the capillary lumen and interfere with blood flow. This stimulates synchronous apoptosis of downstream endothelial cells ('secondary apoptosis') and ultimately obliteration of the vasculature. Removal of the apoptotic vessels is achieved by hyalocytes.

A better understanding of this phenomenon may provide insights into new ways to induce the regression of pathologic angiogenesis or inhibit neovascularization in such conditions as proliferative diabetic retinopathy and exudative age-related macular degeneration. Indeed, the recently developed synthetic vascular endothelial growth factor inhibitors seem to be of limited usefulness in treating pathologic neovascularization in exudative age-related macular degeneration. However, this or a superior inhibitory mechanism may prove to be useful in other proliferative retinopathies, such as retinopathy of prematurity.

Vitreous Imaging

Previously considered a vestigial organ, vitreous is now regarded as an important ocular structure [8, 9], at least with respect to several important pathologic conditions of the posterior segment. This remarkable tissue is in essence an extended extracellular matrix, composed largely of water with a very small amount of structural macromolecules [9, 10]. Nevertheless, in the normal state it is a solid and clear gel, especially in youth (fig. 1). Because of the predominance of water within vitreous, effective imaging of this structure in vitro is best performed by methods that overcome the intended transparency of this tissue yet avoid dehydration. Imaging vitreous in vivo is likely best achieved by visualizing the macroscopic features via an assessment of the nature and organization of the molecular components. The following will review some of the most important methods available for imaging vitreous in vitro and in vivo.

In vitro Imaging

Arguably the best available technique for the histologic characterization of vitreous structure was developed by Faulborn. Through an arduous process of tissue preparation that very slowly dehydrates specimens over months, this technique minimizes the disruption of vitreous structure that results from the rapid dehydration that is induced by standard histologic tissue processing. The elegant preparations obtained with such slow dehydration have provided great insight into the role of vitreous in the pathophysiology of proliferative diabetic vitreoretinopathy [22] (fig. 3) and retinal tears [36] (fig. 4).

Dark-field slit microscopy of whole human vitreous in the fresh, unfixed state was extensively employed by Sebag and Balazs [37] to characterize the fibrous structure of vitreous (fig. 5), age-related changes within the central vitreous body [38] and at the

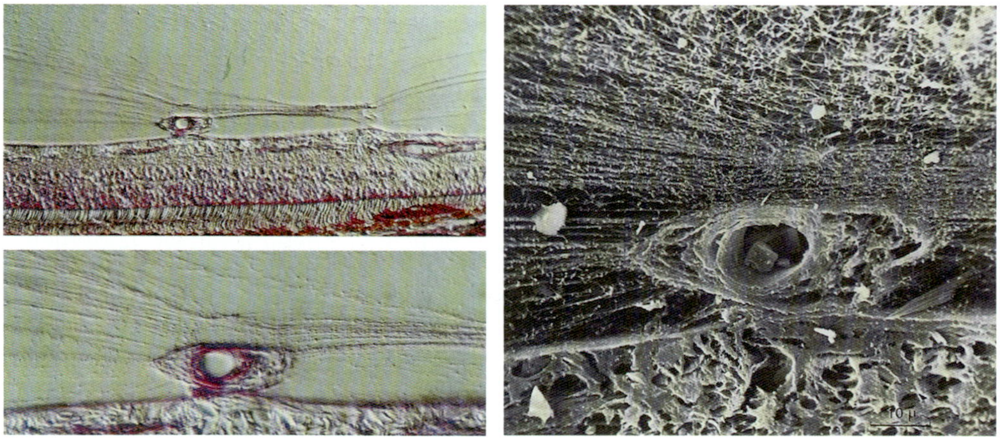

a b c

Fig. 3. Proliferative diabetic vitreoretinopathy. Neovascularization which arises from the disk and retina involves vascular endothelial cell migration and proliferation onto and into the posterior vitreous cortex. These photomicrographs demonstrate the formation of neovascular complexes sprouting into the posterior vitreous cortex of a human eye (bar = 10 μm). Reprinted with permission from Faulborn and Bowald [22].

vitreoretinal interface [39], and the effects of diabetes on human vitreous structure [40]. This imaging method has clearly demonstrated the fibers in the anterior peripheral vitreous (fig. 6) that transmit traction to the peripheral retina in rhegmatogenous retinal pathology. Fibers in this region also play a role in the formation of the so-called 'anterior loop' configuration of anterior proliferative vitreoretinopathy (fig. 7). Traction mediated by this anterior loop causes ciliary body detachment (sometimes with hypotony) and iris retraction in severe cases.

In vivo Imaging

Conventional Ophthalmoscopy and Biomicroscopy

Of all the parts of the eye that are routinely evaluated by physical examination, vitreous is perhaps the least amenable to standard inspection techniques. This is because examining vitreous is an attempt to visualize a structure designed to be virtually invisible [42]. With the direct ophthalmoscope light rays emanating from a point in the patient's fundus emerge as a parallel beam which is focused on the observer's retina and an image is formed. However, incident light reaches only the part of the fundus onto which the image of the light source falls and only light from the fundus area onto which the observer's pupil is imaged reaches that pupil. Thus, the fundus can be seen only where the observed and the illuminated areas overlap and where the light source and the observer's pupil are aligned optically. This restricts the extent of

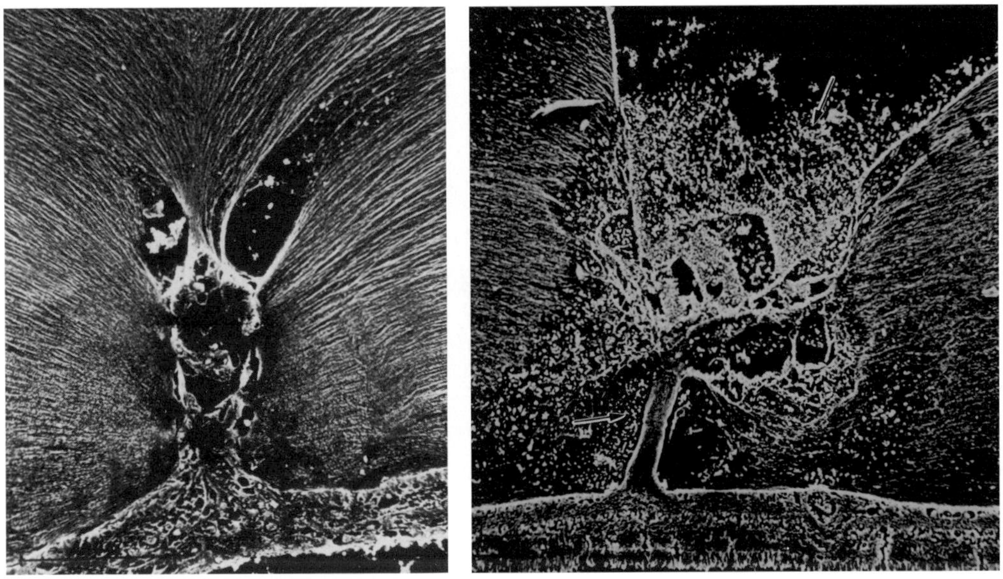

a b

Fig. 4. Morphology of peripheral vitreous. **a** Cystic retinal tuft. The tuft is a cystoid formation of fibers, similar to those of the nerve fiber layer, and cells, similar to those found in the inner plexiform layer of the retina. The tuft is connected to the ILL of the retina. This scanning electron micrograph shows the insertion of the vitreous collagen fibers on the tuft's apical surface. Their orientation changes toward the tuft's surface. Reprinted with permission from Dunker et al. [36]. **b** Verruca. The verruca has a structure similar to that of a tree. Its 'roots' are embedded in the inner layers of the retina. Cellular elements resembling cells of the inner plexiform layer can be seen near the retinal surface. The 'trunk' of this structure extends from the retina to the middle parts of the vitreous cortex. The 'branches' of the verruca are intertwined with interrupted vitreous collagen fibers. Local condensation of collagen fibers exists as well as local collagen destruction (arrows) and interruption of the ILL of the retina. Reprinted with permission Dunker et al. [36].

the examined area and also because of a limited depth of field, this method is rarely used to assess vitreous structure.

Indirect ophthalmoscopy was one of the major contributions of Charles Schepens to the world. It extends the field of view by using an intermediate lens to gather rays of light from a wider area of the fundus. While this technique has been invaluable in the diagnosis and treatment of various vitreoretinal disorders, its use in vitreous alone has been more limited. This is due to the fact that although binocularity provides stereopsis, the image size is considerably smaller than with direct ophthalmoscopy and only significant alterations in vitreous structure, such as a hole in the prepapillary posterior vitreous cortex, vitreous hemorrhage, or asteroid hyalosis, are reliably diagnosed by indirect ophthalmoscopy. The most difficult clinical entity to assess is that of PVD, particularly when anomalous.

Effectively using slit lamp biomicroscopy to overcome vitreous transparency necessitates maximizing the Tyndall effect. Although this can be achieved in vitro, as

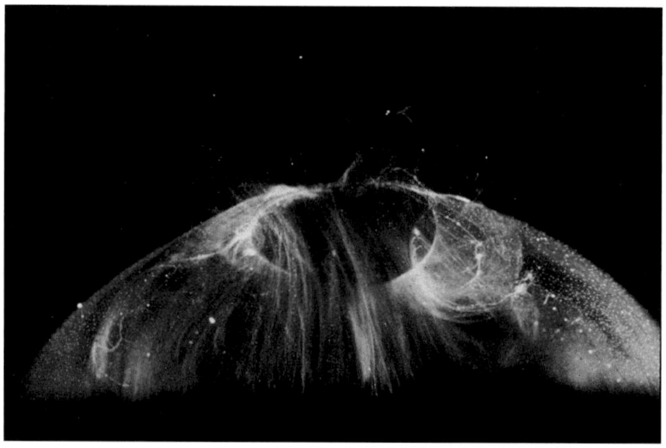

Fig. 5. Posterior and central vitreous of a 59-year-old man. The premacular hole is to the top at the center. Fibers course anteroposteriorly in the center of the vitreous and enter the retrocortical (preretinal) space via the premacular region of the vitreous cortex. Within the cortex are many small 'dots' that scatter light intensely. The larger, irregular dots are debris. The small dots are hyalocytes.

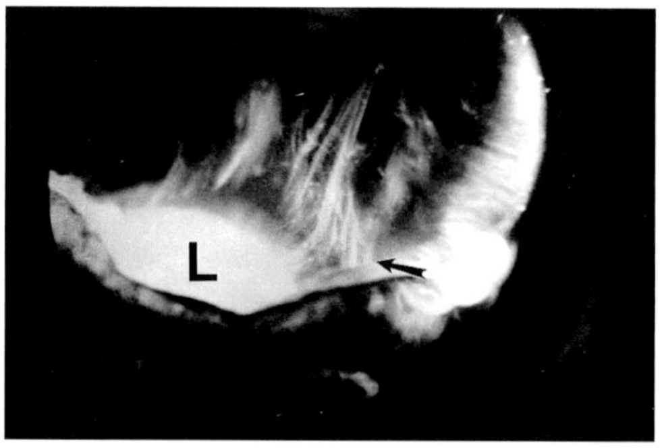

Fig. 6. Vitreous base morphology. Vitreous structure in a 58-year-old female. Fibers course anteroposteriorly in the central and peripheral vitreous. Posteriorly, fibers orient to the premacular region. Anteriorly, the fibers 'splay out' to enter into the vitreous base (arrow). L = Crystalline lens.

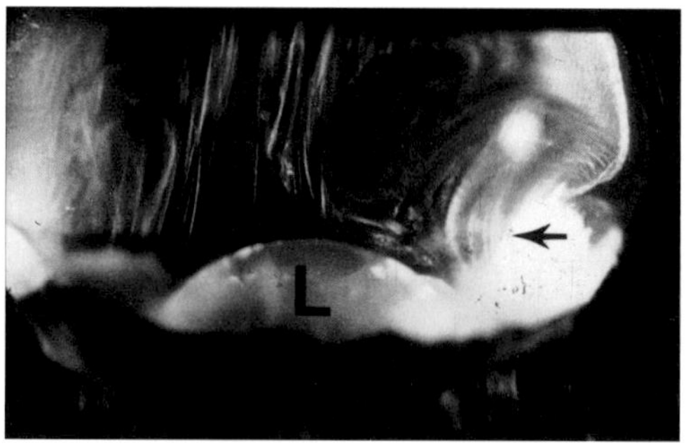

Fig. 7. Vitreous base 'anterior loop'. Central and peripheral vitreous structure in a 76-year-old male. The posterior aspect of the lens is seen below. Fibers course anteroposteriorly in the central vitreous and enter at the vitreous base. The 'anterior loop' configuration at the vitreous base is seen on the right side of the specimen. L = Lens; arrow = anterior loop of vitreous base. Reprinted with permission from Sebag and Balazs EA [41].

described above, there are limitations to the illumination/observation angle that can be achieved clinically. This is even more troublesome in the presence of meiosis, corneal and/or lenticular opacities, and limited patient cooperation. Essential to the success of achieving an adequate Tyndall effect are maximizing pupil dilation in the

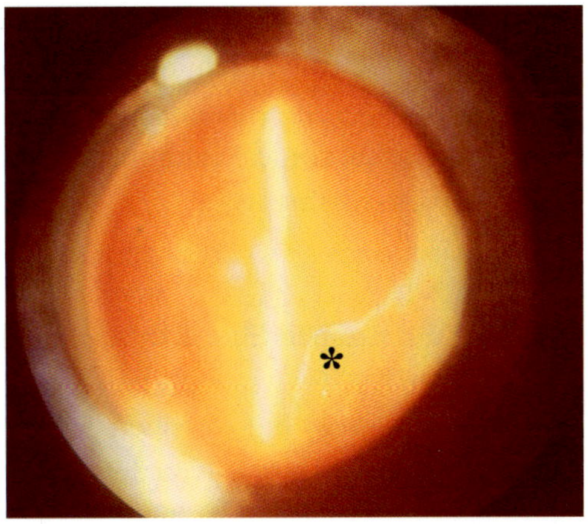

Fig. 8. Fundus photograph of PVD. The detached posterior vitreous cortex (asterisk) can be seen anterior to the optic disk (to the left). Courtesy of Clement Trempe, MD.

patient, since the Tyndall effect increases with an increasingly subtended angle between the plane of illumination and the line of observation (up to a maximum of 90°), and dark adaptation in the examiner. Some observers purport that green light enhances the Tyndall effect, although this has never been explained or tested scientifically. Preset lens biomicroscopy attempts to increase the available illumination-observation angle, offers dynamic inspection of vitreous in vivo, and provides the capability of recording the findings in real time [43]. Initially introduced on a wide scale for use with a Hruby lens and currently practiced by using a hand-held 90-diopter lens at the slit lamp, this technique is purportedly best performed with a fundus camera and the El Bayadi-Kajiura lens promoted by Schepens et al. [43] (fig. 8). This approach has been used in many seminal studies of the role of vitreous in various disease states. However, there has not been widespread use of this approach, probably because it is heavily dependent upon subjective interpretation of the findings and questionable reproducibility from center to center.

Scanning Laser Ophthalmoscopy

The scanning laser ophthalmoscope was developed at the Schepens Eye Research Institute in Boston to enable dynamic inspection of vitreous in vivo. Scanning laser ophthalmoscopy (SLO) features tremendous depth of field, and offers real-time recording of findings. Monochromatic green, as well as other wavelengths of light are also available for illumination [44]. SLO has improved our ability to visualize details in the prepapillary posterior vitreous, such as Weiss's ring. Unfortunately, in spite of the dramatic depth of field possible with this technique, SLO does not adequately image the entire vitreous body and, in particular, the attached posterior vitreous cortex, probably because its thickness is below the SLO level of resolution. Thus, PVD, by far the most common diagnosis to be entertained when imaging vitreous clinically, is not reliably identified by SLO. Indeed, there is an increasing awareness among vitreous surgeons that the reliability of the clinical diagnosis of total PVD by any existing technique is woefully inadequate. This awareness arises from the fact that vitreous surgery following clinical examination often reveals findings that are contradictory to preoperative assessments.

Ultrasonography

Ultrasound is an inaudible acoustic wave that has a frequency of more than 20 kHz. The frequencies used in ophthalmology are generally in the range of 8–10 MHz. Although these very high frequencies produce wavelengths as short as 0.2 mm, these are not short enough to adequately assess normal internal vitreous structure such as the fibers described above. Even the posterior vitreous cortex, about 100 μm at its thickest point in the normal state, is below the level of resolution of conventional ultrasonography. The utility of this technique results from the fact that strong echoes are produced at 'acoustic' interfaces found at the junctions of media with different densities and sound velocities, and the greater the difference in density between the two media that create the acoustic interface, the more prominent the echo. Thus, age-related or pathologic phase alterations within the vitreous body are detectable by ultrasonography.

In the late 1950s and early 1960s, Oksala was among the first to employ B-scan ultrasonography to image vitreous. The findings of his extensive study of aging changes were summarized in 1978 [45]. In that report of 444 'normal' subjects, Oksala defined the presence of acoustic interfaces within the vitreous body as evidence of vitreous aging and determined that the incidence of such interfaces was 5% between the ages of 21–40 years, and fully 80% in individuals over 60 years of age. In clinical practice, however, only profound entities such as asteroid hyalosis, vitreous hemorrhage, and intravitreal foreign bodies (if sufficiently large) are imaged by ultrasonography.

At the vitreoretinal interface, the presence of a PVD is often suspected on the basis of B-scan ultrasonography but can never be definitively established, since the level of resolution of ultrasound is not sufficient to reliably image the posterior vitreous cortex, which is only a little more than 100 μm at its thickest portion. In essence, while the presence of PVD can often be reliably established by ultrasound, its absence cannot. Clinical studies [46] have successfully used this technique to determine that in patients with proliferative diabetic vitreoretinopathy [47], there is a split in the posterior vitreous cortex, called vitreoschisis (fig. 9). The success achieved in using ultrasound to identify this important pathologic entity probably results from the fact that this tissue is abnormally thickened by nonenzymatic glycation of vitreous collagen and other proteins [49]. When not thickened, and indeed when vitreoschisis in non-diabetic patients causes the posterior vitreous cortex to be thinner than normal, the thickness of these tissue planes falls below the level of resolution of this imaging modality.

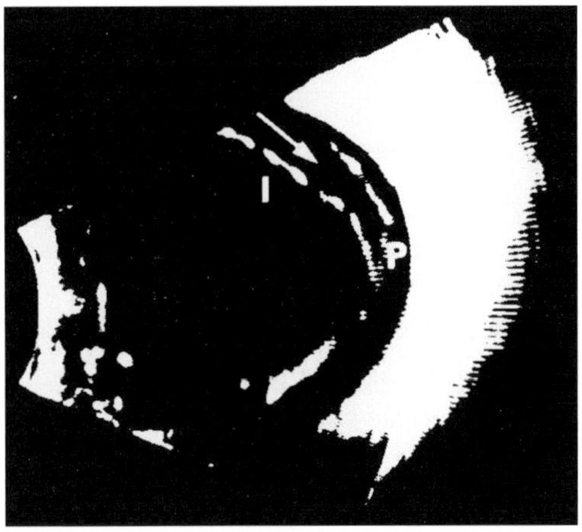

Fig. 9. Ultrasonography imaging of vitreoschisis. Splitting of the vitreous cortex (arrow) can occur and mimic PVD. In diabetic patients, blood can be present in the vitreoschisis cavity. When the blood cells settle to the bottom of the vitreoschisis cavity, a 'boat-shaped' preretinal hemorrhage can result. I = Inner wall; P = posterior wall of the vitreoschisis cavity within the posterior vitreous cortex. Photograph courtesy of Dr. Ronald Green. Reprinted with permission from Green and Byrne [48].

Optical Coherence Tomography

Invented by Fujimoto at MIT and introduced into clinical practice in 1991, optical coherence tomography (OCT) is a new technique for cross-sectional imaging of ocular structures [50]. OCT is based on the principle of low-coherence interferometry, where the distances between and sizes of structures in the eye are determined by measuring the time it takes for light to backscatter from structures at varied axial distances. The resolution of all 'echo'-based imaging technologies (such as ultrasound and OCT) is based upon the ratio of the speed of the incident wave to that of the reflected wave. As described above, vitreoretinal ultrasonography is usually performed with a frequency of 10 MegaHz and has a 150-mm resolution. Although recently introduced ultrasound biomicroscopy has increased the frequency (up to 100 MegaHz), and thus has a spatial resolution of 20 μm, penetration into the eye is no more than 4–5 mm. Light-based devices, such as the OCT, use an incident wavelength of 800 nm and have increased axial resolution to 10 μm, providing excellent imaging of retinal architecture. The limitations of OCT include the inability to obtain high-quality images through media opacities such as dense cataract or vitreous hemorrhage. Furthermore, much of the vitreous body is not presently imaged by OCT, limiting the utility of this technique for vitreous imaging.

To date, OCT has primarily been used to image, and to some extent quantitate, structure and pathologies in the retina, subretinal space, retinal pigment epithelium, and choroid. Vitreous applications that have been useful involve imaging the vitreomacular interface in patients with macular pucker, vitreomacular traction syndrome, diabetic macular edema, and macular holes [51]. Often, however, the exact nature and molecular composition of these preretinal tissue planes cannot be definitively deduced using conventional time domain OCT.

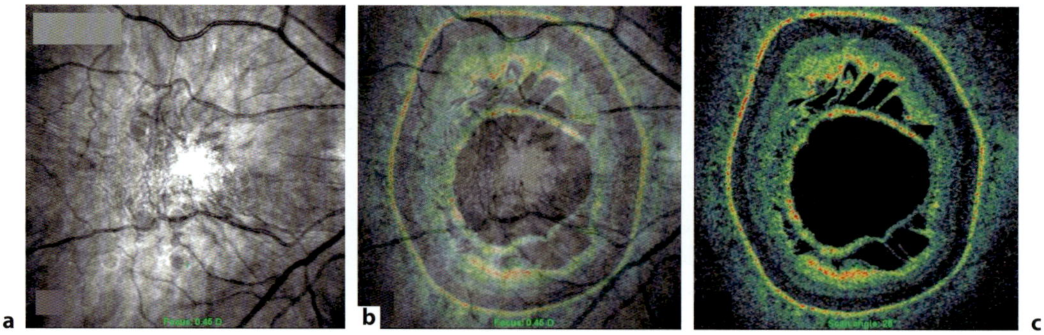

Fig. 10. Coronal plane imaging with combined OCT-SLO. The SLO grayscale fundus image (**a**) overlaid upon the coronal OCT color image (**c**) results in a superimposed image (**b**) used to identify the number of retinal contraction centers in macular pucker.

Combined OCT-SLO

Combined OCT-SLO imaging (OPKO, Inc., Miami, Fla., USA) is a new imaging technology that consists of a dual channel system incorporating an interferometer and a confocal receiver. A broadband infrared superluminescent diode with a wavelength of 820 nm provides the light source. In the longitudinal mode, the OCT-SLO projects light through a Galvano scanning mirror system, moving the beam in a horizontal line to create cross-sectional images of the retina. In the coronal imaging mode (created by transverse scanning), the light is projected through 2 x-/y-plane Galvano scanners moving the beam in a raster fashion across the surface of the retina. Each coronal plane image that is produced is an x-/y-image at a different z-axis depth. The depth resolution is approximately 10 μm while the transverse resolution is approximately 20 μm. For both the coronal and longitudinal OCT scans, a matching grayscale confocal fundus image is also produced. The grayscale SLO confocal fundus image (fig. 10a) and the threshold color OCT image in the coronal plane (fig. 10c) can be superimposed (fig. 10b). There is pixel-to-pixel registration between the two images (coronal OCT and SLO) since they are obtained simultaneously using parallel detector systems. The superimposed coronal plane images are especially useful for identifying centers of retinal contraction in macular pucker, defined as an area where radially oriented retinal striations converge. This feature has also been used to identify the presence of retinal contraction in patients with macular holes.

Coronal plane OCT-SLO imaging studies [52] in 44 patients with macular pucker found multiple foci of retinal contraction and pucker in 20 of the 44 patients (45.5%). Table 1 demonstrates the distribution of the number of pucker centers as identified by SLO-OCT imaging in the coronal plane.

Two distinct foci of retinal contraction (fig. 11b) were detected in 11/44 patients (25%), 3 different sites (fig. 11c) were identified in 5/44 patients (11.4%), and 4/44 (9.1%) had 4 centers of retinal contraction (fig. 11d). Intraretinal cysts were present

Table 1. Stratification of pucker centers demonstrates that nearly half of all membranes (20/44 = 45.5%) have more than one retinal contraction center

Number of retinal contraction centers	One	Two	Three	Four
Number of patients	24	11	5	4
Patient population, %	54.5	25.0	11.4	9.1

in 10/35 (28.6%) subjects with 1 or 2 pucker centers as compared to 6/9 (66.7%) subjects with 3 or 4 centers ($p = 0.05$, Fisher's exact test). The average macular thickness of subjects with 1 or 2 pucker centers was 297 ± 110 versus 369 ± 98 μm for subjects with 3 or 4 pucker centers ($p = 0.05$, t test assuming equal variance). Thus, coronal plane imaging with combined OCT-SLO technology revealed multifocality in macular pucker that has clinical significance. Since eyes with multiple retinal contraction centers had intraretinal cysts twice as frequently, and greater retinal thickening as compared to eyes with only 1 or 2 contraction centers, this may not only impact upon prognosis, but management as well, in that eyes with multiple contraction centers may need to undergo surgery sooner than unifocal cases.

Combined OCT-SLO also enables visualization of the intersecting planes of fundus imaging by SLO in the x-/y-plane, and by OCT in the z-plane (fig. 12). This manufacturer-provided 3-dimensional rendering of the intersection between a longitudinal OCT scan and the SLO image can be used to identify a variety of abnormalities, particularly those that are difficult to visualize, such as vitreopapillary traction, or the centers of an area of retinal contraction in multifocal macular pucker. The SLO fundus images with superimposed coronal plane OCT scans can be analyzed quantitatively with Adobe PhotoShop software, an approach that has proven very useful for quantitative analysis of vitreoretinal topography in macular pucker [55].

In a study [56] of 25 patients with macular holes, OCT-SLO found eccentric macular pucker in 40% of cases. This would have been difficult, if not impossible, to reliably visualize with conventional OCT. Further analysis [57] revealed that when compared to eyes with unifocal macular pucker and no macular holes, the eccentric pucker in patients with macular holes had an average surface area of contraction of 23.12 ± 18.8 mm^2 that was significantly smaller than in macular pucker eyes (63.2 ± 23.7 mm^2; $p = 0.006$). Also, the distance from the center of retinal contraction to the center of the macula was significantly greater in macular hole eyes (8.64 ± 2.33 mm) than macular pucker eyes (4.45 ± 1.9 mm; $p = 0.0001$).

High-resolution time domain OCT-SLO and the newer spectral domain imaging technologies have provided even more powerful methods with which to evaluate the vitreoretinal interface. As a result, new concepts of disease pathogenesis are evolving. For example, vitreoschisis, defined as a split in the posterior vitreous cortex, has pre-

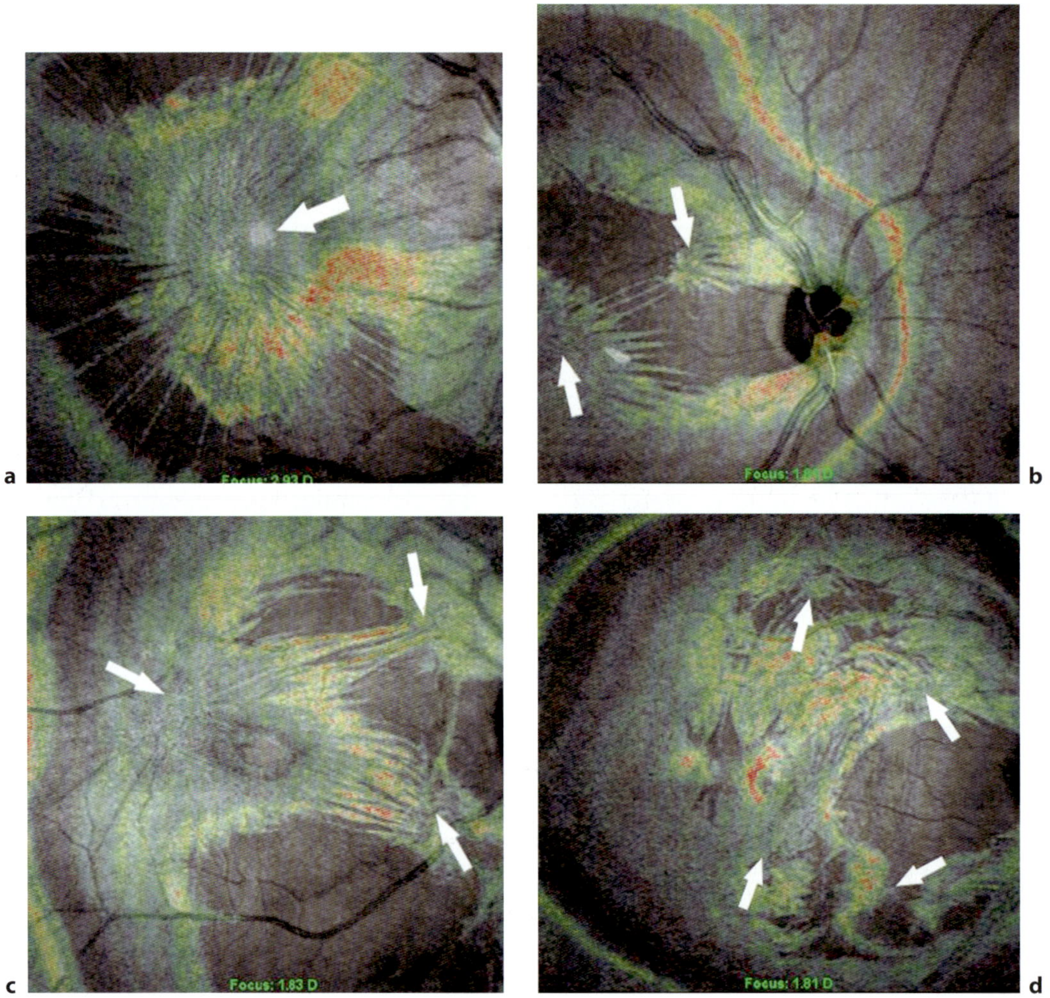

Fig. 11. Coronal plane imaging of macular pucker with combined OCT-SLO. Superimposing coronal plane OCT color images upon the SLO grayscale fundus image reveals multifocality (arrows) in the topography of macular pucker. **a** 1 pucker (retinal contraction) center. **b** 2 centers. **c** 3 centers. **d** 4 centers.

viously been described in proliferative diabetic vitreoretinopathy [47] by ultrasound [46]. However, high-resolution time domain OCT-SLO can better detect this condition in proliferative diabetic vitreoretinopathy than ultrasound (fig. 13). Moreover, studies [57] with high-resolution time domain OCT-SLO have detected vitreoschisis in 24/45 eyes (53.3%) with macular holes, and in 19/44 (43.2%) with macular pucker. Anomalous PVD may be the inciting event in each of these conditions [58]. However, as mentioned above, the topographic and structural features that were detected in eyes with macular holes and eccentric retinal contraction differed in comparison to eyes with macular pucker alone [57], suggesting that while each condition may begin

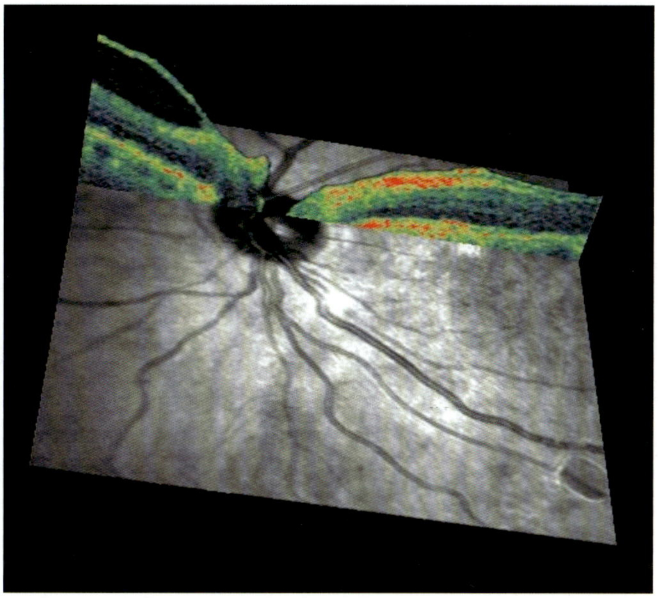

Fig. 12. Three-dimensional OCT-SLO Imaging of vitreopapillary traction. The color OCT image can be intersected with the grayscale SLO fundus image to detect exactly where on the fundus an OCT finding is located. In this eye there is obvious insertion of a vitreous membrane onto the optic disk. In some cases, this can induce optic nerve dysfunction [53]. Vitrectomy can eliminate this form of anomalous PVD [58], with improvements in visual function [54].

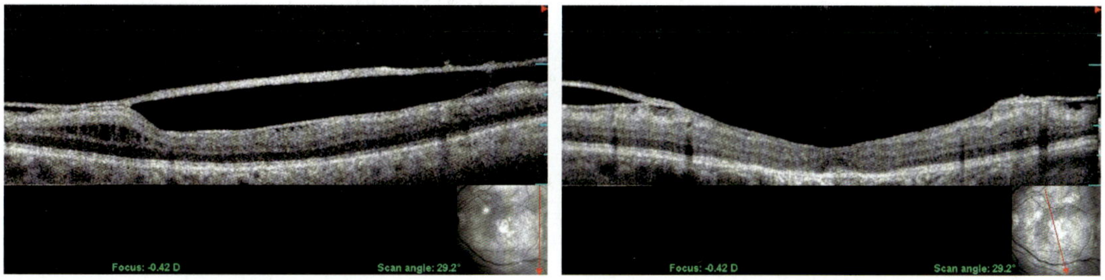

Fig. 13. OCT-SLO imaging of vitreoschisis in proliferative diabetic vitreoretinopathy. A split in the posterior vitreous cortex is visible (arrowhead) on combined OCT-SLO transverse imaging. Significant retinal traction is induced at the point where the two layers of the split posterior vitreous cortex rejoin to form a full-thickness cortex. Often, this is the site of traction retinal detachment.

with anomalous PVD, differences in subsequent cell migration and proliferation probably result in the different clinical appearances. The considerable detail that is afforded by spectral domain imaging will very likely shed more light upon this and other questions.

It is important to note, however, that in spite of the high resolution provided by these imaging technologies, they are still only evaluating changes at the tissue level [59]. Much earlier in the natural history of the disease there are molecular and physiological changes that eventually result in the subsequent cellular and tissue changes. If we are ever to develop preventative therapies, future diagnostic technologies will need to de obtained that can assess ocular health and deviations from this state of health on a molecular and physiologic level. The following presents some of the approaches that are currently in development.

Spectroscopy

Nuclear Magnetic Resonance Spectroscopy. The nuclear magnetic resonance (NMR) spectroscopy phenomenon is based upon the fact that when placed in a magnetic field, nuclei (especially water protons) orient their magnetic vectors along the direction of the magnetic field. The time constant for this orientation, known as the longitudinal relaxation time T_1, reflects the thermal interactions of protons with their molecular environment. Magnetic vectors that have previously been induced to be in phase with each other undergo a 'dephasing' relaxation process that is measured by the transverse relaxation time T_2. It is the transverse relaxation time T_2 that reflects inhomogeneities within the population of protons. Protons oriented by a magnetic field absorb radio waves of the appropriate frequency to induce transactions between their two orientations. Such absorption is the basis of the NMR signal used to index relaxation times. Relaxation times in biologic tissues vary with the concentration and mobility of water within the tissue. As the latter is influenced by the interaction of water molecules with macromolecules in the tissue, this noninvasive measure can assess the gel-to-liquid transformation that occurs in vitreous during aging [38] and disease states, such as diabetic vitreopathy [47, 60]. These considerations led Aguayo et al. [61] to use NMR spectroscopy in studying the effects of pharmacologic vitreolysis [62] of bovine and human vitreous specimens and intact bovine eyes in vitro. Collagenase induced measurable vitreous liquefaction more than hyaluronidase. Thus, this noninvasive method could be used to evaluate age- and disease-induced synchisis (liquefaction) of the vitreous body, although it is not clear whether this technique adequately evaluates the vitreoretinal interface. More recently, NMR spectroscopy has been employed in studies of retinal structure [63] or the measurement of vitreous oxygen as an index of retinal oxygen metabolism [64, 65]. Pilot clinical studies [66] have also attempted to use this technology to index a diabetes-induced breakdown of the blood-retinal barrier. Curiously, few recent studies have investigated intrinsic vitreous structure using this imaging technology.

Raman Spectroscopy. This form of spectroscopy was first described in 1928 by C.V. Raman in India. Raman spectroscopy is an inelastic light scattering technique wherein the vibrational-mode molecules in the study specimen absorb energy from incident photons, causing a downward frequency shift, which is called the Raman shift. Because the signal is relatively weak, current techniques employ laser-induced stimulation with gradual increases in the wavelength of the stimulating laser, so as to be able to detect the points at which the Raman signal becomes apparent as peaks superimposed on the broad background fluorescence. The wavelengths at which these peaks are elicited are characteristic of the chemical bonds, such as aliphatic C—H (2,939 cm^{-1}), water O—H (3,350 cm^{-1}), C═C and C—H stretching vibrations in π-conjugated and aromatic molecules (1,604 cm^{-1} and 3,057 cm^{-1}). To date, most applications of this technique in the eye have been for analysis of lens structure and pathology [67]. The use of near-infrared excitation wavelengths is particularly effective in the lens, since these wavelengths have better penetration into opacified lenses with cataracts.

The first vitreous Raman spectroscopy studies [68] employed excised human vitrectomy samples obtained during surgery. The near-infrared excitation at 1,064 nm was provided by a diode-pumped Nd:YAG CW laser with a diameter of 0.1 mm and a power setting of 300 mW. Backscattering geometry with an optical lens collected scattered light which was passed through a Rayleigh light rejection filter into a spectrophotometer. The results showed that this technique was able to detect peaks at 1,604 cm^{-1} and 3,057 cm^{-1} in vitreous of diabetic patients that were not present in controls. Further research and development is needed to refine the methodology for use in situ, and eventually in vivo, with the ultimate aim of providing a noninvasive technique to assess the tissue effects of diabetes as an adjunct to monitoring blood glucose levels. Not only would this provide another evaluation of diabetes effects on the eye, but might also enable the use of the eye as a window to the body, since these phenomena are ubiquitous.

Recent studies have used Raman spectroscopy to detect the presence of β-carotene in vitreous that was removed at surgery for asteroid hyalosis [69]. Another application of Raman spectroscopy has been to detect intravitreal glutamate levels in vitro [70]. While this approach does not provide information about vitreous anatomy and physiology, it does have potential as a noninvasive way to evaluate intraocular physiology in diabetic retinopathy and glaucoma.

Dynamic Light Scattering

Dynamic light scattering (DLS) is an established laboratory technique to measure the average size (or size distribution) of microscopic particles as small as 3 nm in diameter that are suspended in a fluid medium where they undergo random brownian motion. Light scattered by a laser beam passing through such a dispersion will have intensity fluctuations in proportion to the brownian motion of the particles, resulting in a constantly fluctuating speckle pattern [71]. This speckle pattern is the result of interference in the light paths and it fluctuates as the particles in the scattering medium undergo random movements on a time scale of ≥ 1 μs due to the collisions between themselves and the fluid molecules (brownian motion). Since the size of the particles influences their brownian motion, analysis of the scattered light intensity yields a distribution of the size(s) of the suspended particles. In dilute dispersions, generally the case in biologic tissues, especially in the eye, light scattered from small particles fluctuates rapidly while light scattered from large particles fluctuates more slowly. Calibration and comparison to standards enables the determination of actual particle sizes. In circumstances where there is an active increase (or decrease) in particle sizes (from nanometers to a few micrometers) and/or an increase (or decrease) in the number or density of suspended particles, the result is an increase in scattered light intensity, or polydispersity, which is a measure of the number of distinct groups of species with different sizes. Thus, a change in scattered light intensity and polydispersity can complement particle size determination.

In the eye, visible light from a laser diode (670 nm, power = 50 μW) is focused into the tissue of interest, and backscattered light is collected for analysis. The detected signal is processed via a digital correlator to yield a time autocorrelation function. For dilute dispersions of spherical particles the slope of the time autocorrelation function provides a quick and accurate determination of the particle's translational diffusion coefficient, which can be related to its size via a Stokes-Einstein equation, provided the viscosity of the suspending fluid, its temperature, and its refractive index are known. For the lens and vitreous, a viscosity of $\eta = 0.8904$ cP, a refractive index of $n = 1.333$, and a temperature of 25°C for in vitro studies and 37°C for in vivo studies were used to determine macromolecule sizes.

Ansari [72] has recently authored an overview of ophthalmic applications of DLS and their current state of development. Most of the work has been done in the lens [73], where studies found that DLS was able to detect and quantify the changes induced in a hyperbaric oxygen model of nuclear cataract [74]. In fact, DLS was more sensitive than Scheimpflug photography in detecting early changes in a cold cataract model [75]. A large cross-sectional clinical study performed at the National Eye Institute has been conducted and the results have been submitted for publication.

DLS of vitreous provides information such as diffusion coefficient, particle size, scattered intensity, and polydispersity (measure of heterogeneity). Early studies determined that with this DLS apparatus bovine [76] and human [77] vitreous exhibit bimodal behavior, consistent with the two-component composition of vitreous (HA and collagen macromolecules). In diabetes, there are considerable changes in vitreous biochemistry [49] that induce structural changes [40] due to the aggregation of vitreous proteins, particularly collagen. DLS was not only able to detect, but also quantify these changes on a molecular level [77]. Thus, with this advanced imaging technology, it might be possible to characterize the molecular effects of diabetes on the eye and indeed use the eye as an index for diabetes effects on the entire body. Detecting and characterizing the molecular effects of diabetes in this noninvasive manner will deepen our understanding of the pathophysiology and enable treatments at a very early stage of disease. Repeat testing can be performed often so as to monitor the response to therapy. Such intervention will likely prevent disease advancement to cellular and tissue levels, and ultimately prevent organ failure.

Pharmacologic vitreolysis [62, 78] is a new approach to vitreoretinal therapeutics. The objective is to alter vitreous biochemistry with the intent of eliminating the contribution of vitreous to retinal disease. Since an innocuous (PVD depends upon both liquefaction of the gel and dehiscence at the vitreoretinal interface, agents are being developed to achieve both of these objectives. Substances that liquefy the gel are called 'liquefactants', while those that alter the vitreoretinal interface are known as 'interfactants' [11]. Since agents such as hyaluronidase (Vitrase®) and perhaps plasmim/microplasmin are predominantly liquefactants, their effects must be monitored closely to prevent untoward effects. This is needed to avoid the inadvertent induction of anomalous PVD [58] that might result from inducing excess or precocious liquefaction before adequate vitreoretinal dehiscence has been created. Thus, noninvasive, reproducible, and rapid diagnostic systems need to be developed that can monitor the process of pharmacologic vitreolysis.

Advancement of the field of pharmacologic vitreolysis would greatly benefit from the development of diagnostic technologies that can enable molecular assessment of the state of the vitreous and changes therein. Studies have shown that DLS can provide useful information regarding various aspects of vitreous biochemistry. This molecular diagnostic methodology was shown to be effective in detecting and quantifying the changes induced by hyaluronidase, collagenase, and microplasmin [79]. Indeed, the use of DLS in studying microplasmin showed that this technique could be very useful in quantifying effects on vitreous diffusion coefficients [80], an important property for both health and disease of the vitreous.

Conclusions

The development of new treatments for the cure or prevention of vitreoretinal diseases requires new insights into the causes and progression of these disorders [81]. No single method presently exists that will enable accurate and reproducible noninvasive imaging of both the vitreous body and the vitreoretinal interface. This impacts significantly upon the ability to assess the effects of aging and disease and, in particular, upon the accuracy of diagnosing posterior vitreous detachment clinically. Moreover, this limitation hinders our ability to adequately evaluate the role of vitreous in vitreoretinal diseases such as retinal detachment, both in general terms and in specific clinical cases.

Today, combining more than one of the aforementioned techniques could provide considerably more information than just one technique. For example, NMR spectroscopy could assess the degree of vitreous liquefaction, DLS could determine the concurrent aggregation of collagen and other macromolecules that occurs during liquefaction, Raman spectroscopy could identify the presence of specific molecular moieties that provide insight into the pathogenesis, while combined OCT-SLO could image the vitreoretinal interface. Hopefully, the future will witness the combination of these and other techniques into a single noninvasive instrument for research and clinical applications.

References

1 Duke-Elder SW: The nature of the vitreous body. Br J Ophthalmol 1930;14(suppl IV):6.

2 Redslob E: Le corps vitre. Soc Fr Ophtalmol Monogr. Paris, Masson, 1932, pp 174–178.

3 Eisner G: Biomicroscopy of the Peripheral Fundus. New York, Springer, 1973.

4 Worst JGF: Cisternal systems of the fully developed vitreous body in the young adult. Trans Ophthalmol Soc UK 1977;97:550–554.

5 Sebag J, Balazs EA: Morphology and ultrastructure of human vitreous fibers. Invest Ophthalmol Vis Sci 1989;30:1867–1871.

6 Kishi S, Shimizu K: Posterior precortical vitreous pocket. Arch Ophthalmol 1990;108:979–982.

7 Sebag J: Letter to the editor. Arch Ophthalmol 1991; 190:1059.

8 Foulds WS: Is your vitreous really necessary? The role of the vitreous in the eye with particular reference to retinal attachment, detachment and the mode of action of vitreous substitutes. Eye 1987;1:641–664.

9 Sebag J: The Vitreous: Structure, Function and Pathobiology. New York, Springer, 1989.

10 Sebag J: Macromolecular structure of vitreous. Prog Polym Sci 1998;23:415–446.

11 Sebag J, Yee KMP: Vitreous – From biochemistry to clinical relevance; in Tasman W, Jaeger EA (eds): Duane's Foundations of Clinical Ophthalmology. Philadelphia, Lippincott, Williams & Wilkins, 2006, vol 1, chapt 16.

12 Bishop PN: Structural macromolecules and supramolecular organisation of the vitreous gel. Prog Retin Eye Res 2000;19:323–344.

13 Balazs EA: Molecular morphology of the vitreous body; in Smelser GK (ed): The Structure of the Eye. New York, Academic Press, 1961, pp 293–310.

14 Sheehan JK, Atkins EDT, Nieduszynski IA: X-Ray diffraction studies on the connective tissue polysaccharides. Two dimensional packing scheme for threefold hyaluronic chains. J Mol Biol 1975;91:153–163.

15 Balazs EA: Functional anatomy of the vitreus; in Duane TD, Jaeger EA (eds): Biomedical Foundations of Ophthalmology. Philadelphia, Harper & Row, 1984, chapt 17, p 14.

16 Seery CM, Davison PF: Collagens of the bovine vitreous. Invest Ophthalmol Vis Sci 1991;32:1540–1550.

17 Mayne R: The eye; in Royce PM, Steinmann B (eds): Connective Tissue and Its Heritable Disorders: Molecular, Genetic, and Medical Aspects. New York, Wiley-Liss, 2001, pp 131–141.

18 Comper WD, Laurent TC: Physiological functions of connective tissue polysaccharides. Physiol Rev 1978;58:255–315.

19 Scott JE, Chen Y, Brass A: Secondary and tertiary structures involving chondroitin and chondroitin sulphate in solution, investigated by rotary shadowing electron microscopy and computer simulation. Eur J Biochem 1992;209:675–680.

20 Mayne R, Brewton RG, Ren Z-H: Vitreous body and zonular apparatus; in Harding JJ (ed): Biochemistry of the Eye. London, Chapman and Hall, 1997, pp 135–143.

21 Sebag J, Hageman GS: Interfaces. Eur J Ophthalmol 2000;10:1–3.

22 Faulborn J, Bowald S: Microproliferations in proliferative diabetic retinopathy and their relation to the vitreous. Graefes Arch Clin Exp Ophthalmol 1985; 223:130–138.

23 Mann I: The vitreous and suspensory ligament of the lens; in Mann I (ed): The Development of the Human Eye. New York, Grune & Stratton, 1964, p 150.

24 Jack RL: Regression of the hyaloid artery system: an ultrastructural analysis. Am J Ophthalmol 1972;74: 261–272.

25 Balazs EA: Fine structure of the developing vitreous. Int Ophthalmol Clin 1975;15:53–63.

26 Gloor BP: Zur Entwicklung des Glaskörpers und der Zonula. 3. Herkunft, Lebenszeit und Ersatz der Glaskörperzellen beim Kaninchen. Graefes Arch Clin Exp Ophthalmol 1973;187:21–44.

27 Balazs EA, Toth LZ, Ozanics V: Cytological studies on the developing vitreous as related to the hyaloid vessel system. Graefes Arch Clin Exp Ophthalmol 1980;213:71–85.

28 Raymond L, Jacobson B: Isolation and identification of stimulatory and inhibiting growth factors in bovine vitreous. Exp Eye Res 1982;34:267–286.

29 Lutty GA, Mello RJ, Chandler C, et al: Regulation of cell growth by vitreous humour. J Cell Sci 1985;76: 53–65.

30 Jacobson B, Dorfman T, Basu PK, et al: Inhibition of vascular endothelial cell growth and trypsin activity by vitreous. Exp Eye Res 1985;41:581–595.

31 Feeney SA, Simpson DA, Gardiner TA, Boyle C, Jamison P, Stitt AW: Role of vascular endothelial growth factor and placental growth factors during retinal vascular development and hyaloid regression. Invest Ophthalmol Vis Sci 2003;44:839–847.

32 Mitchell CA, Risau W, Drexler HC: Regression of vessels in the tunica vasculosa lentis is initiated by coordinated endothelial apoptosis: a role for vascular endothelial growth factor as a survival factor for endothelium. Dev Dyn 1998;213:322–333.

33 Ito M, Yoshioka M: Regression of the hyaloid vessels and papillary membrane of the mouse. Anat Embryol 1999;200:403–411.

34 McMenamin PG, Djano J, Wealthall R, Griffin BJ: Characterization of the macrophages associated with the tunica vasculosa lentis of the rat eye. Invest Ophthalmol Vis Sci 2002;43:2076–2082.

35 Meeson A, Palmer M, Calfon M, Lang R: A relationship between apoptosis and flow during programmed capillary regression is revealed by vital analysis. Development 1996;122:3929–3938.

36 Dunker S, Glinz J, Faulborn J: Morphologic studies of the peripheral vitreoretinal interface in humans reveal structures implicated in the pathogenesis of retinal tears. Retina 1997;17:124–130.

37 Sebag J, Balazs EA: Human vitreous fibres and vitreoretinal disease. Trans Ophthalmol Soc UK 1985; 104:123–128.

38 Sebag J: Age-related changes in human vitreous structure. Graefes Arch Clin Exp Ophthalmol 1987; 225:89–93.

39 Sebag J: Age-related differences in the human vitreoretinal interface. Arch Ophthalmol 1991;109:966–971.

40 Sebag J: Abnormalities of human vitreous structure in diabetes. Graefes Arch Clin Exp Ophthalmol 1993;231:257–260.

41 Sebag J, Balazs EA: Pathogenesis of cystoid macular edema: an anatomic consideration of vitreoretinal adhesions. Surv Ophthalmol 1984;28(suppl): 493–498.

42 Sebag J: Classifying posterior vitreous detachment – A new way to look at the invisible. Br J Ophthalmol 1997;81:521–522.

43 Schepens CL, Trempe CL, Takahashi M: Atlas of Vitreous Biomicroscopy. Boston, Butterworth Heinemann, 1999.

44 Mainster MA, Timberlake GT, Webb RH, Hughes GW: Scanning laser ophthalmoscopy – Clinical applications. Ophthalmology 1982;89:852–857.

45 Oksala A: Ultrasonic findings in the vitreous body at various ages. Albrecht Von Graefes Arch Klin Exp Ophthalmol 1978;207:275–280.

46 Chu T, Lopez PF, Cano MR, Green RL: Posterior vitreoschisis – An echographic finding in proliferative diabetic retinopathy. Ophthalmology 1996;103: 315–322.

47 Kroll P, Rodrigues E, Hoerle S: Pathogenesis and classification of proliferative diabetic vitreoretinopathy. Ophthalmologica 2007;221:78–94.

48 Green RL, Byrne SF: Diagnostic ophthalmic ultrasound; in Ryan SJ (ed): Retina. St Louis, Mosby, 1989.

49 Sebag J, Buckingham B, Charles MA, Reiser K: Biochemical abnormalities in vitreous of humans with proliferative diabetic retinopathy. Arch Ophthalmol 1992;110:1472–1479.

50 Fujimoto JG, Brezinski ME, Tearney GJ, et al: Optical biopsy and imaging using optical coherence tomography. Nat Med 1995;1:970–972.

51 Srinivasan VJ, Wojtkowski M, Witkin AJ, Duker JS, Ko TH, Carvalho M, Schuman JS, Kowalczyk A, Fujimoto JG: High-definition and 3-dimensional imaging of macular pathologies with high-speed ultrahigh-resolution optical coherence tomography. Ophthalmology 2006;113:2054e1–2054e14.

52 Gupta P, Sadun AA, Sebag J: Multifocal retinal contraction in macular pucker analyzed by combined optical coherence tomography/scanning laser ophthalmoscopy. Retina 2008;28:447–452.

53 Kroll P, Wiegand W, Schmidt J: Vitreopapillary traction in proliferative diabetic vitreorctinopathy. Br J Ophthalmol 1999;83:261–264.

54 Meyer CH, Schmidt JC, Mennel S, Kroll P: Functional and anatomical results of vitreopapillary traction after vitrectomy. Acta Ophthalmol Scand 2007; 85:221–222.

55 Gupta P, Christofferson S, Sadun AA, Sebag J: Quantitative Analysis of Premacular Membranes with Pucker Using Scanning Laser Ophthalmoscope/ Optical Coherence Tomography (SLO-OCT) Imaging. Fort Lauderdale, ARVO, 2007.

56 Sebag J, Rosen RR, Garcia P, et al: Coronal plane imaging with combined OCT-SLO detects macular pucker in macular holes. Meet Club Jules Gonin, Cape Town, 2006.

57 Sebag J, Gupta P, Rosen RR, Garcia P, Sadun AA: Macular holes and macular pucker: The role of vitreoschisis as imaged by optical coherence tomography/scanning laser ophthalmoscopy. Trans Am Ophthalmol Soc 2007;105:121–131.

58 Sebag J: Anomalous PVD – A unifying concept in vitreo-retinal diseases. Graefes Arch Clin Exp Ophthalmol 2004;242:690–698.

59 Sebag J, Ansari RR: Ophthalmic diagnostics. J Biomed Opt 2004;9:8.

60 Sebag J: Diabetic vitreopathy. Ophthalmology 1996; 103:205–206.

61 Aguayo J, Glaser B, Mildvan A, et al: Study of vitreous liquefaction by NMR spectroscopy and imaging. Invest Ophthalmol Vis Sci 1985;26:692–697.

62 Sebag J: Pharmacologic vitreolysis. Retina 1998;18: 1–3.

63 Cheng H, Nair G, Walker TA, Kim MK, Pardue MT, Thulé PM, Olson DE, Duong TQ: Structural and functional MRI reveals multiple retinal layers. Proc Natl Acad Sci USA 2006;103:17525–17530.

64 Zaharchuk G, Busse RF, Rosenthal G, Manley GT, Glenn OA, Dillon WP: Noninvasive oxygen partial pressure measurement of human body fluids in vivo using magnetic resonance imaging. Acta Radiol 2006;13:1016–1024.

65 Ngumah QC, Buchthal SD, Dacheux RF: Longitudinal non-invasive proton NMR spectroscopy measurement of vitreous lactate in a rabbit model of ocular hypertension. Exp Eye Res 2006;83:390–400.
66 Trick GL, Liggett J, Levy J, Adamsons I, Edwards P, Desai U, Tofts PS, Berkowitz BA: Dynamic contrast enhanced MRI in patients with diabetic macular edema: initial results. Exp Eye Res 2005;81:97–102.
67 Nie S, Bergbauer KL, Kuck JFR Jr, Yu NT: Near infrared Fourier transform Raman spectroscopy in human lens research. Exp Eye Res 1990;51:619–623.
68 Sebag J, Nie S, Reiser KA, Charles MA, Yu NT: Raman spectroscopy of human vitreous in proliferative diabetic retinopathy. Invest Ophthalmol Vis Sci 1994;35:2976–2980.
69 Lin SY, Chen KH, Cheng WT, Ho CT, Wang SL: Preliminary identification of Beta-carotene in the vitreous asteroid bodies by micro-Raman spectroscopy and HPLC analysis. Microsc Microanal 2007;13:128–132.
70 Katz A, Kruger EF, Minko G, Liu CH, Rosen RB, Alfano RR: Detection of glutamate in the eye by Raman spectroscopy. J Biomed Opt 2003;8:167–172.
71 Chu B: Laser Light Scattering: Basic Principles and Practice. New York, Academic Press, 1991.
72 Ansari RR: Ocular static and dynamic light scattering: a non-invasive diagnostic tool for eye research and clinical practice. J Biomed Opt 2004;9:46–57.
73 Datiles MB, Ansari RR, Reed GF: A clinical study of the human lens with a dynamic light scattering device. Exp Eye Res 2002;74:93–102.
74 Simpanya MF, Ansari RR, Suh KI, Leverenz VR, Giblin FJ: Aggregation of lens crystallins in an in vivo hyperbaric oxygen guinea pig model of nuclear cataract: dynamic light scattering and HPLC analysis. Invest Ophthalmol Vis Sci 2005;46:4641–4651.
75 Ansari RR, Datiles MB: Use of dynamic light scattering and Scheimpflug imaging for the early detection of cataracts. Diabetes Technol Ther 1999;1: 159–168.
76 Ansari RR, Dunker S, Suh K, Kitaya N, Sebag J: Quantitative molecular characterization of bovine vitreous and lens with non-invasive dynamic light scattering. Exp Eye Res 2001;73:859–866.
77 Sebag J, Ansari RR, Dunker S, Suh SI: Dynamic light scattering of diabetic vitreopathy. Diabetes Technol Ther 1999;1:169–176.
78 Sebag J: Is pharmacologic vitreolysis brewing? Retina 2002;22:1–3.
79 Sebag J: Molecular biology of pharmacologic vitreolysis. Trans Am Ophthalmol Soc 2005;103: 473–494.
80 Sebag J, Ansari RR, Suh KI: Pharmacologic vitreolysis with microplasmin increases vitreous diffusion coefficients. Graefes Arch Clin Exp Ophthalmol 2007;245:576–580.
81 Kroll P: New insights into the diagnosis and treatment of vitreoretinal diseases. Ophthalmologica 2007;221:215.

J. Sebag, MD
7677 Center Avenue
Huntington Beach, CA 92647 (USA)
Tel. +1 714 901 7777, Fax +1 714 901 7770, E-Mail jsebag@VMRinstitute.com

Meyer CH (ed): Vital Dyes in Vitreoretinal Surgery.
Dev Ophthalmol. Basel, Karger, 2008, vol 42, pp 29–34

Historical Aspects and Evolution of the Application of Vital Dyes in Vitreoretinal Surgery and Chromovitrectomy

Eduardo B. Rodrigues[a] · Fernando M. Penha[a] · Bruno Furlani[a] · Carsten H. Meyer[b] · Mauricio Maia[a] · Michel E. Farah[a]

[a]Vision Institute, Department of Ophthalmology, Federal University of Sao Paulo, Sao Paulo, Brazil; [b]Department of Ophthalmology, University of Bonn, Bonn, Germany

Abstract

Lobeck and coworkers performed the first intravitreal application of vital dyes to visualize preretinal structures in 1932. Since then numerous investigators in the 20th century examined the use of biological stains through the endovenous, subretinal and intravitreal delivery route in order to identify vitreoretinal tissues and breaks. However, in the year 2000, a new surgical approach, recently coined *chromovitrectomy,* has arisen, which consists in the intraoperative application of vital dyes during vitrectomy. Initially fluorescein, and more recently indocyanine green, trypan blue, bromophenol blue, triamcinolone acetonide and patent blue have been used for the staining of preretinal membranes and tissues. Currently, many vital stains are under evaluation in animals for future clinical application during chromovitrectomy such as indigo carmine or light green. In this paper, several historical considerations in regard to the application of vital dyes in chromovitrectomy are discussed.

Historically, the development of dyes and evidence of selective affinity of biological tissues for certain dyes had remarkable effects upon ancient and modern medicine. For instance, in the 19th century, the Spanish neuroanatomist Santiago Ramón y Cajal used chemical dyes to define discrete physiologic and abnormal areas of the brain. The father of immunology and pioneer of chemotherapy, Paul Ehrlich, demonstrated fascination with the affinity of dyes for tissues and the underlying chemistry of the reaction which would later prove pivotal in leading the formulation of some fundamental principles of immunology. More recently in modern medicine, radiologists found contrast agents very useful for the in vivo enhancement of human healthy and diseased tissues, whereas gastroenterologists, oncologists and neurosurgeons routinely apply intraoperative vital dyes to identify transparent tumors, inflammation, or scarred tissues [1].

In ophthalmology, vital dyes have long been used as diagnostic aids. Fluorescein dye may be placed on the corneal surface to identify denuded epithelial-free areas in corneal epithelial defects, while rose bengal may stain cellular remnants and debris of damaged epithelial cells [2]. In the retinal diagnostic field, sodium fluorescein and indocyanine green dyes may be injected endovenously for observation and contrast of chorioretinal vessels and tissues. Recently, vital dyes have been used in ophthalmic surgery in order to enable surgeons to better visualize the semitransparent intraocular membranes and tissues [3]. For vitreoretinal surgery, there are currently a variety of targeted tissues which may be highlighted by selective vital dyes including the vitreous, internal limiting membrane (ILM) and epiretinal membrane [4]. This paper presents the historical evolution of the use of vital dyes in the surgical treatment of vitreoretinal diseases and its implication for a modern technique, herein named chromovitrectomy.

Early Experiments with Endovenous Application of Dyes in Vitreoretinal Surgery

One of the first reports on the use of biological stains for retina surgery described the endovenous route of administration. In 1939, Sorsby [5] reported the clinical application of vital dyes for the visualization of retinal tears in the therapy of rhegmatogenous retinal detachments. He endovenously applied Kiton fast green V in a few patients with retinal detachment, and observed a greenish appearance of the detached retina, which provided a fine distinction with the unstained retinal break. Later, Offret and Decaudin [6] in 1950 and Simonelli and Faldi [7] in 1953 injected fluorescein also through the endovenous route and described a 'good visibility' as the retinal tear was separated from the pale retina by a colored edge. In 1966, Eisner [8] published the findings of a new additional phenomenon, i.e. the flow of the dye from the subretinal space towards the subhyaloidal space after endovenous application, while, in 1968, Jütte and Lemke [9] found out that those previous observations occurred only in light-pigmented retinas from Caucasians and myopic patients. For this and other reasons this approach has not gained popularity for the purpose of staining retinal tissue in the surgical treatment of rhegmatogenous retinal detachment. Nevertheless, the endovenous route for the injection of indocyanine green and fluorescein became the gold standard for the diagnostic staining of the retinal and choroidal vessels during angiography (table 1).

Early Experiments with Intravitreal and Subretinal Injection of Dyes in Vitreoretinal Surgery

In 1932, Lobeck [10] and coworkers were the first to perform intravitreal injection of vital dyes; they applied India ink in animals. Interestingly, just a couple of hours later

Table 1. Stains tested during vitreoretinal surgery before vitrectomy

Surgeon	Year	Stain	Route of administration	Indication – surgical pearl
Lobeck	1932	India ink	intravitreal	choroid important for drainage of subretinal fluid
Sorsby	1939	fast green	endovenous	good retinal break visualization
Hruby	1946	methylene blue	subretinal	not aware of subretinal drainage of fluid
Black	1947	methylene blue	subretinal	claiming that subretinal route potentially toxic
Offret	1950	fluorescein	endovenous	good retinal break visualization
Simonelli	1953	fluorescein	endovenous	good retinal break visualization
Niedermeier	1964	Evans blue	intravitreal	path of dye passes through retinal break
Eisner	1966	fluorescein	endovenous	inward dye flow into subhyaloid space
Jütte	1968	fluorescein	endovenous	no dye contrast in pigmented retinas
Kutschera	1969	various	intravitreal	patent blue least toxic

the regions of retinal breaks and choroidal capillaries were brightly colored. Such observations enabled the understanding of the choroidal role for the drainage of intraocular liquids. Three decades later, in 1964, Niedermeier [11] intravitreally injected Evans blue in animal experiments and noticed that a path of dye passed through the retinal break in patients with retinal detachment. In 1969, Kutschera [12] claimed that India ink could induce retina toxicity; therefore, he performed experiments to look for safer vital dyes for intravitreal application and recognition of retinal breaks, vitreous and preretinal contractive tissues in retinal detachment surgery. In this work, Kutschera conducted research in order to determine the safest and most appropriate vital dye to provide the contrast between the colored retinal surface and unstained retinal hole. His results demonstrated that benzopurpurine 4B, trypan red and Chicago blue as well as trypan blue induced a prolonged and too bright vitreous and optic nerve coloring that impaired retinal view. Kutschera [12] concluded that patent blue showed best coloring properties and systemic safety for the retina by analyzing the retinal metabolism in rabbits after endovenous patent blue injection, and by observing neither histologic nor clinical damage to the retinal and vitreous tissue metabolism after exposure to patent blue. He also concluded that vitreous elimination occurred 48 h after the dye injection. These results would later provide important laboratory data for the clinical application of patent blue for chromovitrectomy [13].

In regard to the subretinal route for dye delivery, Black [14] postulated in 1947 that subretinal dye injection could enable better visualization of retinal breaks in retinal detachment surgery. Black aspirated a bit of subretinal fluid after injection of 0.3 ml of liquid methylene blue 0.1% into the subretinal fluid through a transscleral needle. The holes in the retina colored as red spots against a blue retina. He limited his experiments to cases of advanced retinal detachment, as he feared the potential dye toxicity to the macular region. In 1946, Hruby [15] in Graz, Austria, also intravitreally injected methylene blue into the subretinal space to visualize retinal breaks. However,

Table 2. Characteristics of present stains in chromovitrectomy

	Fluorescein	Indocyanine green	Infracyanine green	Trypan blue
Chemical formula	$C_{20}H_{10}Na_2O_5$	$C_{43}H_{47}N_2NaO_6S_2$	$C_{43}H_{47}N_2NaO_6S_2$	$C_{34}H_{24}N_6Na_4O_{14}S_4$
Molecular weight Da	376	774	774	961
Chemical group	xanthene	tricarbocyanine	tricarbocyanine	diazo
Color	red-brownish	dark green	dark green	dark blue
Introduction in chromovitrectomy	1978	2000	2002	2003

he was not aware of the physiologic flow of the vitreous toward the subretinal space, so that the dye was absorbed by the retinal pigment epithelium. Therefore, he reported these experiments as unsuccessful (table 1).

Current Intraoperative Staining of Preretinal Membranes during the Vitreoretinal Surgery 'Chromovitrectomy'

Chromovitrectomy was motivated by the difficulty in visualizing several thin and transparent tissues in the vitreoretinal interface such as the ILM, epiretinal membrane or vitreous, particularly, the posterior hyaloid membrane. A pioneer report has been released by Abrams et al. [16] demonstrating the first intraoperative use of vital dye during vitreoretinal surgery, with fluorescein as a good adjuvant for vitreous identification. Interestingly, this technique remained dormant for several decades until recent years. However, since 2000 the application of dyes to stain preretinal tissues during vitreoretinal surgery, *chromovitrectomy*, has become a widely spread technique among vitreoretinal surgeons. The intravitreal injection of indocyanine green facilitated the visualization of the fine and transparent ILM [17]. Later, trypan blue has been proposed as a helpful tool to identify the several epiretinal membranes, and the intravitreal steroid triamcinolone acetonide was found to stain the vitreous [18]. Recently, few other dyes including infracyanine green, patent blue, bromophenol blue, brilliant blue and sodium fluorescein have been proposed as alternative dyes during chromovitrectomy [19]. Detailed information regarding their use in chromovitrectomy will be reviewed by other papers in this book (table 2).

Final Remarks

Experiments with vital dyes in the early 20th century may have given some evidence for their current use in chromovitrectomy. For example, the experiments by Niedermeier

Triamcinolone	Patent blue	Bromophenol blue	Fluorometholone	Brilliant blue
$C_{24}H_{31}FO_6$	$C_{27}H_{31}N_2NaO_6S_2$	$C_{19}H_{10}Br_4O_5S$	$C_{24}H_{31}FO_5$	$C_{47}H_{48}N_3S_2O_7Na$
434	582	670	418	854
long-acting steroid	triarylmethane	triarylmethane	steroid	triarylmethane
white	blue	dark blue	white	blue
2003	2006	2006	2007	2006

[11] and Kutschera [12] provided the scientific basis for recent research with patent blue in the last few years, which ultimately turned into the marketed dye product named Blueron® (Geuder, Germany). The experiments by Sorsby [5] as early as 1939 with endovenous fast green injection revealed a fine coloring of the retinal surface. Interestingly, some of our preliminary data in animals have shown that intravitreal fast green may induce no retinal toxicity and promotes significant ILM staining, thereby arising as an outstanding alternative stain for chromovitrectomy [unpublished data]. Subretinal application of trypan blue for intraoperative visualization of retinal breaks has recently been demonstrated in the clinical setting in humans [20]. The outstanding work by Kutschera [12] in 1969 compared few vital stains, and found patent blue superior – in regard to staining properties and safety – in comparison to trypan blue. Similarly, our working group also demonstrated a slightly safer profile of patent blue over trypan blue in the rabbit animal model of retina toxicity [21]. In summary, previous experiments from the early and mid 20th century enabled novel thoughts and perspectives for dye application in chromovitrectomy, a widely spread surgical approach in modern vitreoretinal surgery.

Acknowledgment

This work has been supported by the Fehr Foundation, Marburg, Germany, the FAPESP-Fundação de Amparo a Pesquisa do Estado de Sao Paulo, and by the PAOF – Pan-American Ophthalmological Foundation.

References

1 Acosta MM, Boyce HW: Chromoendoscopy – Where is it useful? J Clin Gastroenterol 1998;27:13–20.
2 Kim J: The use of vital dyes in corneal disease. Curr Opin Ophthalmol 2000;11:241–247.
3 Fritz WL: Fluorescein blue, light-assisted capsulorhexis for mature or hypermature cataract. J Cataract Refract Surg 1998;24:19–20.
4 Rodrigues EB, Meyer CH, Kroll P: Chromovitrectomy: a new field in vitreoretinal surgery. Graefes Arch Clin Exp Ophthalmol 2005;243:291–293.

5 Sorsby A: Vital staining of the fundus. Trans Ophthal Soc UK 1939;59:727–730.
6 Offret G, Decaudin A: La fluorescein permet-elle d'aider a la mise en evidence de certaines lesions de la rétine ? Bull Soc Ophthalmol Fr 1950;2:66–70.
7 Simonelli M, Faldi S: Su una migliore visibilita delle rotture retiniche dopo iniezione endovenosa di coloranti vitali. G Ital Oftalmol 1953;6:322–329.
8 Eisner G: Spaltlamenuntersuchungen der hinteren Augenabschnitte nach intravenöser Fluoreszeininjektion. Ophthalmologica 1966;152:396–401.
9 Jütte A, Lemke L: Intravital staining of the fundus oculi with fluorescein sodium. Buch Augenarzt 1968; 49:1–128.
10 Lobeck E: Untersuchungen über die Bedeutung des Netzhautrisses bei Netzhautablösung. Experimentelle Untersuchungen über den intraocularen Flüssigkeitswechsel bei künstlicher Netzhautablösung. Albrecht Von Graefes Arch Ophthalmol 1932;128: 513–573.
11 Niedermeier S: Tierexperimenteller Untersuchungen zur Frage chorioretinaler Gefässstörungen nach Netzhautlochentstehung. Studie zur Pathogenese und Heilung der Amotio Retinae. Albrecht Von Graefes Arch Ophthalmol 1964;167:201–207.
12 Kutschera E: Vital staining of the detached retina with retinal breaks. Albrecht Von Graefes Arch Klin Exp Ophthalmol 1969;178:72–87.
13 Hiebl W, Gunther B, Meinert H: Substances for staining biological tissues: use of dyes in ophthalmology. Klin Monatsbl Augenheilkd 2005;222: 309–311.
14 Black GW: Some aspects of the treatment of simple detachment of the retina, including vital staining of the retina by methylene blue. Trans Ophthalmol Soc UK 1947;67:313–322.
15 Hruby K: Neuere Untersuchungsergebnisse zur Klinik und Pathologie des Glaskörpers. Wien Klin Wochenschr 1946;58:461–469.
16 Abrams GW, Topping T, Machemer R: An improved method for practice vitrectomy. Arch Ophthalmol 1978;96:521–525.
17 Rodrigues EB, Meyer CH, Farah ME, Kroll P: Intravitreal staining of the internal limiting membrane using indocyanine green in the treatment of macular holes. Ophthalmologica 2005;219:251–262.
18 Wong KL, Hiscott P, Stanga P, et al: Trypan blue staining of the internal limiting membrane and epiretinal membrane during vitrectomy: visual results and histopathological findings. Br J Ophthalmol 2003; 87:216–219.
19 Rodrigues EB, Meyer CH, Maia M, Penha FM, Dib E, Farah ME: Vital dyes for chromovitrectomy. Curr Opin Ophthalmol 2007;18:179–187.
20 Jackson TL, Kwan AS, Laidlaw AH, Aylward W: Identification of retinal breaks using subretinal trypan blue injection. Ophthalmology 2007;11:241–247.
21 Maia M, Penha FM, Rodrigues EB, Príncipe A, Dib E, Meyer CH, Freymuller E, Moraes N, Farah ME: Effects of subretinal injection of patent blue and trypan blue in rabbits. Curr Eye Res 2007;32:309–317.

Eduardo B. Rodrigues, MD
Rua Presidente Coutinho 579, conj 501
Florianópolis, SC 88015–300 (Brazil)
Tel./Fax +55 48 3222 3380, E-Mail edubrodriguess@yahoo.com.br

Meyer CH (ed): Vital Dyes in Vitreoretinal Surgery.
Dev Ophthalmol. Basel, Karger, 2008, vol 42, pp 35–42

Three Simple Approaches to Visualize the Transparent Vitreous Cortex during Vitreoretinal Surgery

Jörg C. Schmidt · Jacques Chofflet · Steffen Hörle · Stefan Mennel · Carsten H. Meyer

Department of Ophthalmology, Philipps-University, Marburg, Germany

Abstract

Background: Initial historical considerations to perform a pars plana vitrectomy were made for opaque vitreous cortex due to dense asteroid hyalosis or vitreous hemorrhages. However, current indications for vitreoretinal surgery include mainly vitrectomies in the presence of a clear vitreous, for example retinal detachments, epiretinal membranes or macular holes, thus visualization of the transparent vitreous gel facilitates proper vitreous removal. **Materials and Methods:** The transparent structure of the vitreous cortex as well as the thin epiretinal membrane may become visible during surgery by mild vitreous hemorrhages or intravitreous application of 0.05 ml crystalline triamcinolone acetonide. Eyes with a significant breakdown of the blood-retinal barrier accumulate intravenously applied vital dyes, for example fluorescein, in the vitreous cavity. **Results:** Mild accidental intraoperative bleedings or intended injection of 0.05 ml autologous blood may help to stain transparent vitreous structures and visualize the remaining vitreous. Intravitreous triamcinolone crystals attach to the surface of the vitreous cortex, bursa premacularis or retina itself allowing better visualization of a controlled vitreous removal. A preoperative diagnostic fluorescein angiography in eyes with active uveitis or diabetic retinopathy may lead to a moderate accumulation of the dye in the vitreous cavity and greenish staining of the vitreous cortex at the vitreoretinal interface. **Discussion:** A safe and complete removal of clear vitreous or transparent membranes may be achieved by the intraoperative application of autologous blood or triamcinolone. The preoperative systemic application of fluorescein greatly enhances the visualization of previously clear structures.

The human vitreous cortex is a transparent gel which allows an unscattered transmission of light to the retina. Opacification of the vitreous gel may lead to visual disturbance and was among the initial historical considerations to perform a pars plana vitrectomy. Kastner was the first to perform an open-sky vitrectomy in a patient with amyloidosis in 1968, and Machemer et al. [1] were the first to describe pars plana vitrectomy using a closed system to remove vitreous hemorrhages and asteroid hyalosis in 1971. After the opaque structures were removed, the deteriorated vision significantly

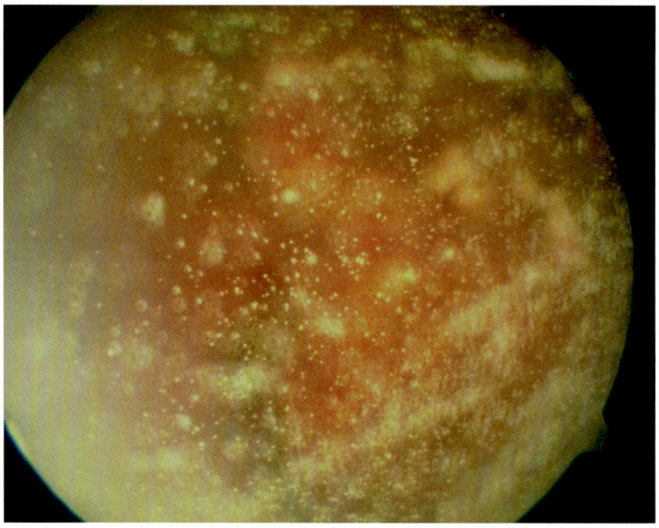

Fig. 1. In asteroid hyalosis, white crystals facilitate visualization of the vitreous.

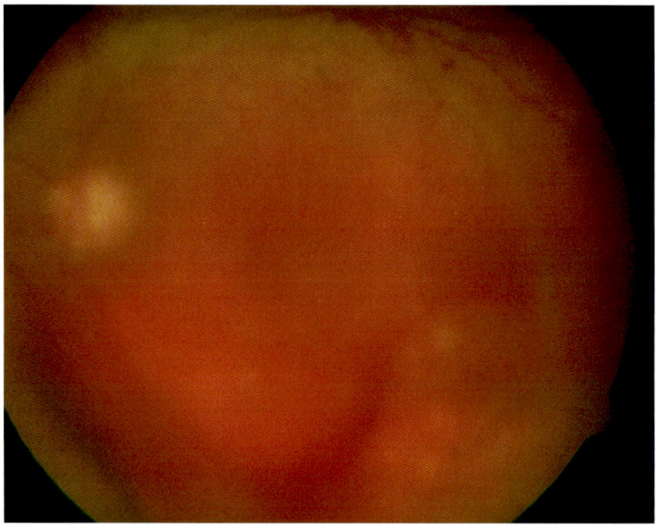

Fig. 2. Blood adhering to the vitreous allows better visualization of the vitreous.

improved [2, 3]. However, current indications for a vitreoretinal surgery include mainly vitrectomies in eyes with a clear vitreous, for example retinal detachments, epiretinal membranes, macular holes or even vitreous floaters [4]. Thus, we need an excellent visualization of the transparent vitreous gel during vitrectomy. Zyvoinović et al. [5] taught us that the vitreous base has to be thoroughly cleaned before silicone oil can be instilled in order to avoid the development of posterior traction or anterior loop

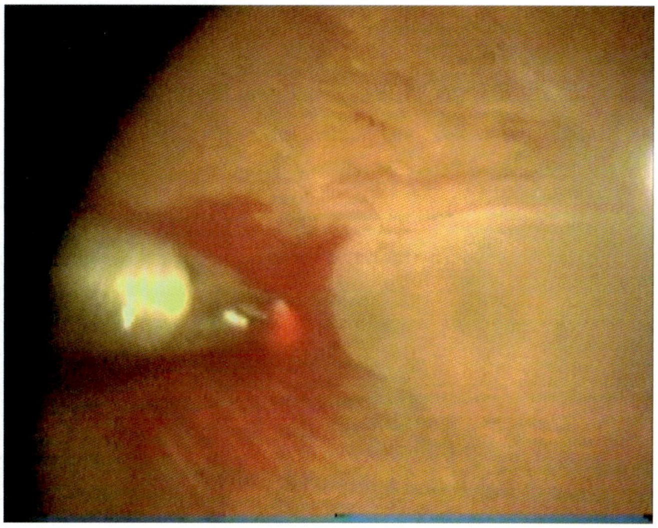

Fig. 3. A fresh hemorrhage at the posterior pole coagulates, settles down onto preretinal membranes and may then be removed together with them.

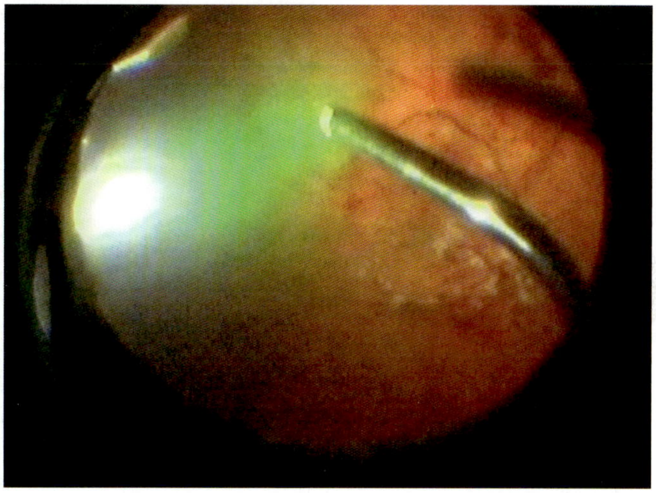

Fig. 4. The vitreous appears greenish 1 day following fluorescein angiography.

formation, leading to redetachment and hypotony. Eckardt et al. [6] advised peeling the internal limiting membrane (ILM) in macular surgery, in order to eliminate all posterior traction and possible diffusion barriers. Unfortunately, these structures are very poorly visible during surgery so that natural stains or vital dyes are currently used to visualize these semitransparent structures.

Fig. 5. Steroid crystals introduced intraoperatively settle onto the posterior vitreous cortex and facilitate visualization of an induced posterior vitreous detachment.

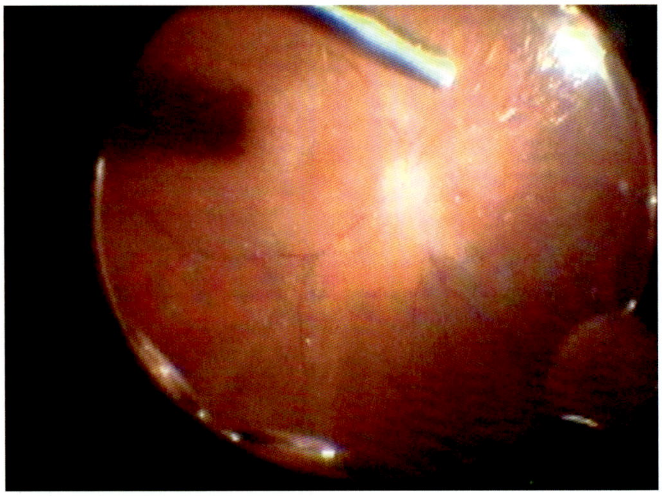

Fig. 6. In this case, steroid crystals sticking to the posterior pole facilitate removal of the ILM at the fovea using a microforceps.

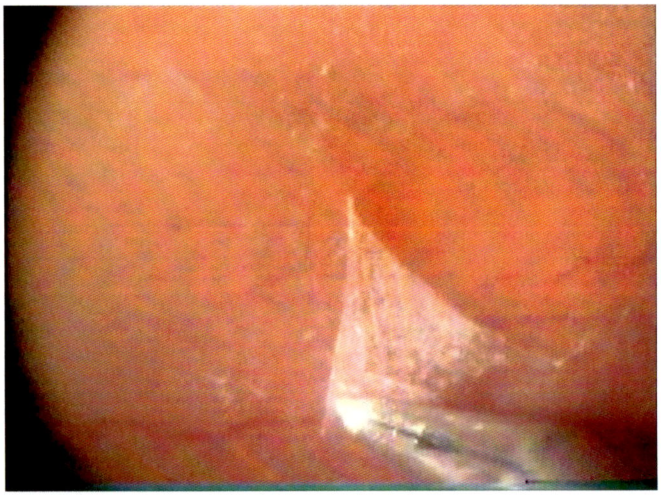

Intravitreous Application of Autologous Blood

When a mild intraoperative vitreous hemorrhage occurs, the freshly liberated blood cells adhere to the collagen net of the clear vitreous, visualizing the three-dimensional structure of the remaining cortex in the vitreous cavity [7, 8]. The reddish staining of the vitreous cortex enhances its visualization as well as complete and controlled removal with a vitreous cutter. Freshly injected autologous erythrocytes also tend to coagulate and settle on the retinal surface. This effect may be used to visualize the

Table 1. Milestones in the treatment with triamcinolone acetonide

Author	Year	Treatment
Schindler et al. [9]	1982	clearance of intravitreous triamcinolone acetonide
Laatikainen and Tarkkanen [10]	1986	management of purulent postoperative endophthalmitis
Jonas et al. [11]	2003	intravitreous injection of crystalline cortisone as adjunctive treatment of proliferative vitreoretinopathy
Peyman et al. [12]	2000	triamcinolone acetonide as an aid to visualize the vitreous and the posterior hyaloid membrane during pars plana vitrectomy
Sakamoto et al. [13]	2002	triamcinolone-assisted pars plana vitrectomy improves the surgical procedures and decreases the postoperative blood-ocular barrier breakdown
Burk et al. [14]	2003	visualizing the vitreous using Kenalog suspension
Matsumoto et al. [15]	2007	triamcinolone acetonide-assisted pars plana vitrectomy improves residual posterior vitreous hyaloid membrane removal: ultrastructural analysis of the ILM

epiretinal membrane during peeling maneuvers in diabetic vitreoretinopathy in a very controlled fashion. However, since fresh blood is not transparent, it is not helpful in the removal of the ILM, because it prevents its delicate three-dimensional visualization.

Intraocular hemorrhages in the elderly tend to accumulate and originate in the inferior quadrant of the vitreous, inducing a posterior vitreous detachment. The posterior vitreous hyaloid membrane may be seen as a sheen-like sheet. However, additional unclotted erythrocytes may become lysed in the meantime and the irrigation fluid swirls the liberated hemoglobin in the vitreous cavity obscuring the view to the fundus by a dusty appearance.

Crystalline Steroids Settle on the Surface of Vitreous Structures

The intravitreous application of triamcinolone acetonide plays an important role in the treatment of numerous vitreoretinal diseases. Its angiostatic and anti-inflammatory effect induces a stabilization of the blood-retinal barrier and permeability of retinal vessels. Suspensions of triamcinolone crystals have also been injected into the vitreous cavity during vitrectomy to visualize intravitreous structures (table 1). Crystalline triamcinolone acetonide may be injected with a 30-gauge cannula into the vitreous cavity after a primary core vitrectomy [16–20]. The swirling white crystals settle unspecifically onto the vitreous surface, epiretinal membranes and retinal surface giving the vitreous cavity the appearance of a 'landscape with first snow'. Thus, the surgical induction or completion of a posterior vitreous detachment becomes easily visible and the complete and safe removal of the posterior vitreous hyaloid membrane can be observed in a controlled fashion. Bursa premacularis or tractional elements at the posterior pole, which have to be removed during macular surgery, may also become visible by triamcinolone crystals. In advanced vitreoretinal surgery, for example macular translocations, a complete peripheral vitreous removal is required to perform a successful surgery and to avoid postoperative traction by membrane formation. If the view becomes obscured in these cases and the complete removal of the vitreous cortex is uncertain, a triamcinolone injection may help to visualize and confirm the status of the complete vitrectomy. Most crystals stick firmly to the surfaces and become only gradually flushed away by the irrigation fluid. However, dense pockets of crystalline deposits on the retinal surface may be gently removed with a suction cannula.

Triamcinolone does not stain the ILM of the retinal surface as specifically as indocyanine green, which has a high affinity for extracellular membranes. However, the assistance of triamcinolone acetonide may be used to visualize the ILM in macular hole surgery when the membrane is not very firmly attached and ILM peeling is easy. But if the ILM itself is very adherent to the retina, as frequently seen in diabetic macular edema, the crystals may be flushed from the surface of the ILM before the membrane is completely removed. These cases may be treated with indocyanine green to ensure a specific staining and complete peeling of the ILM. Some triamcinolone crystals, remaining in the vitreous cavity at the end of surgery, are welcome as a small-dose intravitreous depot to reduce early postoperative inflammation.

Preoperative Fluorescein Angiography May Stain the Vitreous Greenish

Eyes with proliferative vitreoretinopathy, uveitis, vasculitis or retinal vein occlusion are frequently associated with a severe breakdown of the inner blood-retinal barrier. Many of the patients receive a fluorescein angiography 1–2 days before vitrectomy to assess the leakage and retinal edema. In 1994, Chofflet and Kroll observed that, after fluorescein angiography, the primarily transparent vitreous cortex stained light green during vitrectomy. The greenish vitreous was illuminated with conventional endo-light sources and could easily be removed. However, fluorescein demonstrated no staining of the epiretinal membrane and therefore was not recommended for this maneuver. A recent paper evaluated the efficacy of orally administered sodium fluorescein to stain the clear vitreous 12–16 h before vitrectomy in patients with proliferative diabetic vitreoretinopathy. The sodium fluorescein concentration in the vitreous samples ranged from 122 to 282.0 ng/ml and the clear vitreous appeared markedly green so that the surgeons could easily differentiate the residual clear vitreous [21].

Discussion

In any surgery, it is very important to visualize and identify the structures which require treatment. The inspection of the vitreous and the posterior hyaloid membrane is frequently easier in elderly people, as the vitreous becomes liquefied, detached from the retinal surface and has a slightly cloudy appearance [22]. The visualization of dense vitreous strands will be further enhanced, if structures are incorporated into the vitreous scaffold, as frequently seen in asteroid hyalosis or slight vitreous hemorrhage. However, the staining of the vitreous should remain transparent so that adjacent structures of the retina can be seen. Dense hemorrhages prevent a backscattering of light from the retina, so that the vitreous cavity appears as a black hole.

However, today many indications for vitrectomy include eyes with a clear vitreous, for example macular holes, macular puckers or cystoid macular edemas. These conditions complicate the visualization of posterior vitreous membranes as well as of the remaining vitreous pockets. Induction of a posterior vitreous detachment, which is the key to surgical success in these cases, is considerably more difficult. Simple steps may be used to achieve a better visualization during surgery. Fluorescein angiography a few days prior to the surgery or a slight vitreous bleeding during surgery lead to an adherence of blood cells to vitreous structures, thus facilitating visualization of the vitreous. If blood samples are taken using vials with citrate or if they have been centrifuged, problems may arise from substances inhibiting coagulation and from a lack of sterility. If membranes are stained with blood, poor transparency of blood impairs visualization of deeper tissues. Blood may coagulate and adhere to the tissue, while anticoagulated blood is easily flushed away. The current discussion about vital dyes suitable for chromovitrectomy should also include autologous cells, pigment or blood, which induce a natural stain of the vitreous. Even for beginners, a posterior vitreous detachment may be reliably visualized and dyes may be avoided in membranectomies, if a steroid crystal suspension is applied. Whether visualization of the vitreous may be enhanced further beyond the greenish appearance of fluorescein by means of special light sources as in angiography will have to be investigated further.

Acknowledgment

This work has been supported by the Fehr Foundation, Marburg, Germany.

References

1 Machemer R, Büttner H, Norton EW, Parel JM: Vitrectomy: a pars plana approach. Trans Am Acad Ophthalmol Otolaryngol 1971;75:813–820.

2 Machemer R: Vitrectomy in the management of severe diabetic retinopathies. Klin Monatsbl Augenheilkd 1973;162:199–205.

3 Treister G, Machemer R: Results of vitrectomy for rare proliferative and hemorrhagic diseases. Am J Ophthalmol 1977;84:394–412.

4 Hörauf H, Müller M, Laqua H: Vitreous body floaters and vitrectomy with full visual acuity. Ophthalmologe 2003;100:639–643.

5 Zivojnović R, Mertens DA, Baarsma GS: Fluid silicon in detachment for surgery. Klin Monatsbl Augenheilkd 1981;179:17–22.

6 Eckardt C, Eckardt U, Groos S, Luciano L, Reale E: Removal of the internal limiting membrane in macular holes. Clinical and morphological findings. Ophthalmologe 1997;94:545–551.

7 Kroll P, Le Mer Y: Treatment of preretinal retrohyaloidal hemorrhage: value of early argon laser photocoagulation. J Fr Ophtalmol 1989;12:61–66.

8 Le Mer Y, Kroll P, Chofflet J, Hesse L: Systematic search of the posterior vitreous cortex during vitrectomy. Technique, complications and results. J Fr Ophtalmol 1994;17:459–464.

9 Schindler RH, Chandler D, Thresher R, Machemer R: The clearance of intravitreal triamcinolone acetonide. Am J Ophthalmol 1982;93:415–417.

10 Laatikainen L, Tarkkanen A: Management of purulent postoperative endophthalmitis. Ophthalmologica 1986; 193:34–38.

11 Jonas JB, Söfker A, Degenring R: Intravitreal triamcinolone acetonide as an additional tool in pars plana vitrectomy for proliferative diabetic retinopathy. Eur J Ophthalmol 2003;13:468–473.

12 Peyman GA, Cheema R, Conway MD, Fang T: Triamcinolone acetonide as an aid to visualization of the vitreous and the posterior hyaloid during pars plana vitrectomy. Retina 2000;20:554–555.

13 Sakamoto T, Miyazaki M, Hisatomi T, Nakamura T, Ueno A, Itaya K, Ishibashi T: Triamcinolone-assisted pars plana vitrectomy improves the surgical procedures and decreases the postoperative blood-ocular barrier breakdown. Graefes Arch Clin Exp Ophthalmol 2002;240:423–429.

14 Burk SE, Da Mata AP, Snyder ME, Schneider S, Osher RH, Cionni RJ: Visualizing vitreous using Kenalog suspension. J Cataract Refract Surg 2003; 29:645–651.

15 Matsumoto H, Yamanaka I, Hisatomi T, Enaida H, Ueno A, Hata Y, Sakamoto T, Ogino N, Ishibashi T: Triamcinolone acetonide-assisted pars plana vitrectomy improves residual posterior vitreous hyaloid removal: ultrastructural analysis of the inner limiting membrane. Retina 2007;27:174–179

16 Robbie SJ, Snead MP: Intravitreal triamcinolone staining observation of residual undetached cortical vitreous after posterior vitreous detachment. Eye 2007; 21:285–286.

17 Chen TY, Yang CM, Liu KR: Intravitreal triamcinolone staining observation of residual undetached cortical vitreous after posterior vitreous detachment. Eye 2006;20:423–427.

18 Yamaguchi T, Inoue M, Ishida S, Shinoda K: Detecting vitreomacular adhesions in eyes with asteroid hyalosis with triamcinolone acetonide. Graefes Arch Clin Exp Ophthalmol 2006;13:1–4.

19 Schalnus R, Ohrloff C: The blood-retina barrier and blood-aqueous humor barrier in type I diabetic patients without retinopathy. Determination of permeability using fluorophotometry and laser flare measurements. Klin Monatsbl Augenheilkd 1993; 202:281–287.

20 Lobo CL, Bernardes RC, Santos FJ, Cunha-Vaz JG: Mapping retinal fluorescein leakage with confocal scanning laser fluorometry of the human vitreous. Arch Ophthalmol 1999;117:631–637.

21 Yao Y, Wang ZJ, Wei SH, Huang YF, Zhang MN: Oral sodium fluorescein to improve visualization of clear vitreous during vitrectomy for proliferative diabetic retinopathy. Clin Experiment Ophthalmol 2007;35:824–827.

22 Walton KA, Meyer CH, Harkrider CJ, Cox TA, Toth CA: Age-related changes in vitreous mobility as measured by video B scan ultrasound. Exp Eye Res 2002;74:173–180.

Prof. Dr. med. Jörg C. Schmidt
Department of Ophthalmology, Philipps-University Marburg
Robert-Koch-Strasse 4
DE–35037 Marburg (Germany)
Tel. +49 6421 286 2600, Fax +49 6421 286 5678, E-Mail jc.schmidt@gmx.de

Meyer CH (ed): Vital Dyes in Vitreoretinal Surgery.
Dev Ophthalmol. Basel, Karger, 2008, vol 42, pp 43–68

Safety Parameters for Indocyanine Green in Vitreoretinal Surgery

Salvatore Grisanti[a,b] · Andreas Altvater[a] · Swaantje Peters[a,b]

[a]Center for Ophthalmology, University Eye Hospital, Eberhard-Karls-University of Tübingen, Tübingen; [b]Department of Ophthalmology, University of Luebeck, Luebeck, Germany

Abstract

Since the early nineties removal of the internal limiting membrane (ILM) has been shown to be an effective and safe treatment option for conditions that involve the vitreoretinal interface. Peeling of the barely visible ILM, however, represents a challenge and complete removal is difficult and not always obvious. Damage at the vitreoretinal interface or unsatisfactory peeling may therefore be the result of the genuine procedure. Introduction of indocyanine green (ICG) for ILM staining led to better visibility of the ILM and greatly facilitated this surgical maneuver making ILM peeling more controllable, easier and faster. Consequently, enthusiastic acceptance resulted in an uncritical use not supported by preclinical safety data. Soon thereafter some clinical reports raised concerns about potential cytotoxic effects related to the intravitreal use of ICG. The following chapter summarizes the results of in vitro, ex vivo, in vivo and clinical studies related to the use of ICG in vitreoretinal surgery. Critical appraisal of the methodical procedures and results leads to the nonnegligible fact that ICG has a cytotoxic effect enhanced by photoactivation. The results of several studies as well as our experimental workup, however, showed that ICG toxicity to the retinal pigment epithelium is dependent on the dye concentration, the osmolarity of the solvent solutions, as well as on the lengths of dye exposure time and of the vitrectomy endolight illumination time. With respect to the safety margins and profile, ICG is therefore a useful surgical tool that is still widely applied, but that may be replaced by more inert and as efficient vital dyes.

Since Kelly and Wendel [1] first reported on the successful closure of macular holes by pars plana vitrectomy with gas-fluid exchange in a pilot study, several modifications and improvements of the surgical technique have been suggested [2–5].

As thorough and complete removal of the internal limiting membrane (ILM) seems to be an important requirement for visual and anatomical success in macular hole surgery [6, 7], introduction of indocyanine green (ICG) as a vital dye to stain the nearly invisible basement membrane was a major technical improvement. Staining the ILM or epiretinal membranes (ERM) allows surgeons to work more quickly and precisely, thereby potentially improving surgical safety and anatomical outcomes.

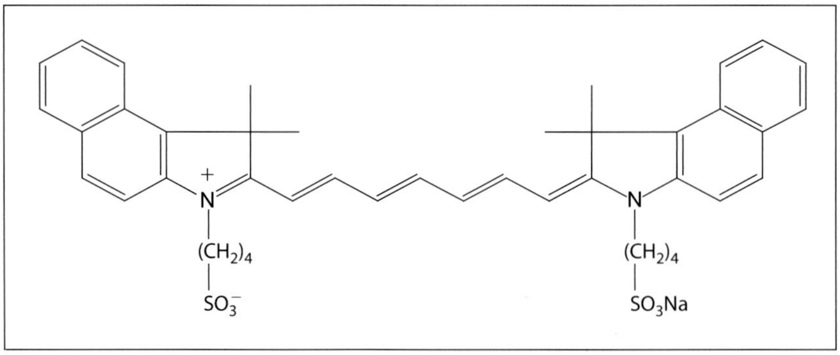

Fig. 1. Chemical formula of ICG.

Indocyanine Green

ICG (fig. 1) is an amphiphilic tricarbocyanine dye which was initially introduced in 1957. It soon became popular for measuring the cardiac output, liver function and for ophthalmic angiography [8–11]. The main advantages were the confinement to the vascular compartment by binding to plasma proteins and the rapid excretion into the bile. Furthermore, it cannot easily permeate living cells with intact cellular membranes [12]. However, it has been shown that absorption properties of ICG exhibit significant variations which depend on the solvent solution and on the concentration used [13, 15]. ICG has little systemic toxicity [16, 17], though there is no information regarding overdosage in humans [18, 19].

ICG was initially introduced to ophthalmology in 1973 to study the choroidal circulation [11]. The dye's capability to bind to basement membranes was first recognized by cataract surgeons and used to improve visualization of the anterior lens capsule for anterior capsulorrhexis in dense white cataract [20]. The main present use of ICG in posterior segment surgery is to facilitate the visualization of the barely visible ILM during macular hole surgery (fig. 2), allowing surgeons to peel more quickly and accurately [21, 22].

The Wrong Way to Go: Clinical Experience without Sufficient Preclinical Data

Since the first report by Grizzard and Tornambe [23] and in numerous following publications, the application of ICG became an eminent tool in facilitating ILM peeling [24–120] during macular surgery. The enthusiasm associated with this controlled and improved technique of ILM peeling led to the widespread use of the dye. As a result of

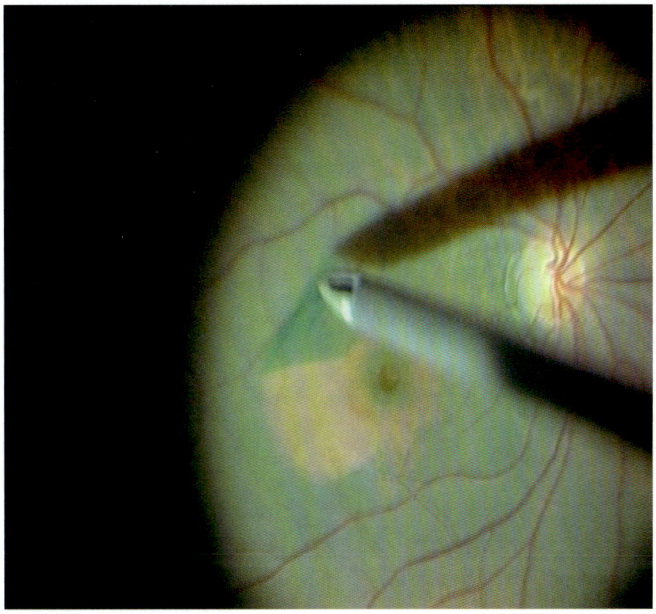

Fig. 2. Intraoperative view of ICG-assisted ILM peeling and the peeled area in macular hole surgery.

gaining experience, about 100 clinical reports using ICG have been published during the past years. Although the majority of these reports retained positive functional and anatomical outcomes, 17 clinical publications (partly from the same group) added to the growing suspicion that intravitreal ICG may be toxic to retinal tissues [29, 31, 54, 63, 65, 66, 69, 73, 90, 91, 93, 95, 101, 102, 107, 114, 119].

So far, no standardized protocol has been used and the surgical techniques as well as volumes, doses and concentrations of ICG were highly variable among the different series. In macular surgery, the concentration of ICG injected into the air- or fluid-filled vitreous ranged from 0.25 to 5.0 mg/ml, and the dye volumes used for ILM staining ranged from 3 drops or 0.1 to 2.0 ml. However, the use of such wide ranges could not explain most of the negative outcomes, and results were partly contradictory as well as indicatory as shown in two previous clinical studies originating from one group [69, 70]. Ando et al. [69] used 0.1–0.2 ml of 5.0 mg/ml ICG (corresponding to doses of 0.5–1.0 mg) and reported unfavorable visual acuity after brief exposure (few seconds) to the dye. However, they revised their previous impression, detecting no difference in the long-term follow-up and comparison of patients receiving ILM peeling with or without ICG [70]. In contrast, Da Mata et al. [101, 110] used 0.3 ml of 5.0 mg/ml ICG (corresponding to a dose of 1.5 mg) and observed no dye-related adverse effects even after an exposure time of 3–5 min. Several investigations similarly reported conflicting results on outcome with an intraocular persistence of ICG up to several months [67, 93, 96, 97, 103, 104, 117].

Regarding these conflicting reports and potential phototoxicity of ICG, various laboratory studies, including animal, ex vivo and in vitro experiments, were performed to understand the effects of ICG [121–173].

Use and Misuse: How to Interpret Preclinical Data

In order to fulfil the prerequisite of clinical practice, experimental in vitro, ex vivo, and in vivo data related to the use of ICG in ophthalmology were collected. These data showed that ICG can be toxic both in vitro and in vivo, supporting already existing knowledge collected in experiments not related to ophthalmology [174–178]. These results were often used by some authors to support their negative clinical experience and to propose the exclusion of ICG from clinical use. Though ICG was demonstrated to be toxic even under certain conditions, neglecting the safety profile of a substance is as wrong as its uncritical use.

The aim of this review is to consider both experimental and clinical studies to confer the safety parameters related to the clinical use of ICG. In order to better understand the ICG-related effects in the context of clinical and experimental practice several parameters are discussed separately.

Clinical Experience and the Experimental Correlate

Reported ICG concentrations range from 0.25 to 5.0 mg/ml when ILM peeling is performed in air- or gas-filled eyes. Lower concentrations are achieved, if ICG staining is performed in fluid-filled eyes under balanced salt solution (BSS). In present clinical practice, volumes of 0.1–0.5 ml are usually applied to the vitreous cavity and left in place for less than 30 s to up to 1 min [69, 75, 76, 89, 91, 95, 98, 99, 105, 111, 114, 116, 118–120, 148, 174].

Da Mata et al. [69] reported that 0.3 ml of ICG at 5.0 mg/ml (corresponding to a dose of 1.5 mg) was a safe and useful adjunct for ILM peeling in macular hole surgery. The dye was left in the vitreous cavity for 3–5 min and removed thereafter by active suction. This technique was based on a preliminary study with human cadaver eyes by the same study group [174]. Sakamoto et al. [179] showed that 0.5 ml of ICG at 5.0 mg/ml (corresponding to a dose of 2.5 mg) was similarly useful for ERM peeling and without any evidence for toxicity. Contrary to these findings, Ando et al. [69] using 0.1–0.2 ml of ICG at 5.0 mg/ml (corresponding to doses of 0.5–1.0 mg) reported on less favorable outcomes and even irreversible peripheral visual field loss when results of ICG-assisted membrane peeling were compared to those without ICG. In contrast, the same study group using ICG at 0.5 mg/ml (corresponding to doses of 0.05–0.1 mg) for ILM staining observed no dye-related adverse effects [70]. In both studies, there was only brief exposure to the dye (around 10 s) and the same volume

Table 1. Median cell survival of ARPE-19 cells after incubation with ICG (0.125–5.0 mg/ml) for 1 min and illumination for 5 min

ICG concentration, mg/ml	Follow-up at 6 h, %		Follow-up at 24 h, %		Follow-up at 72 h, %	
	median	CI	median	CI	median	CI
ICG 5.0	89.87	87.62–91.92	78.34	75.33–81.20	70.22	66.91–73.43
ICG 2.5	95.92	94.40–97.22	94.41	92.67–95.94	91.63	89.55–93.50
ICG 1.0	100.00	100.00–100.00	100.00	100.00–100.00	99.10	98.30–99.65
ICG 0.125	100.00	100.00–100.00	99.88	99.50–100.00	99.89	99.52–100.00

CI = Confidence interval.

was applied. Thus, according to this study ICG at 5.0 mg/ml appeared to be toxic and ICG-related toxicity seemed to be concentration dependent even at exposure times below 1 min. The results of the study by Ando et al. [69] are consistent with a recent experimental workup we performed. In the clinical setup of our study, we tried to mimic the situation that occurs in clinical practice. We used 0.1 ml of ICG at 5.0 mg/ml (corresponding to a dose of 0.5 mg) for 1 min coupled with 5 min of illumination using a standard vitrectomy endolight pipe. We noticed a significant decrease in retinal pigment epithelial cell viability (90% cell survival after 6 and 70% after 72 h of follow-up) and an increase in morphologic change (12% morphologically altered cells after 6 and 28% after 72 h of follow-up) compared to lower-concentrated ICG solutions and the dye-free controls (table 1; fig. 3).

In addition to clinical investigations in air- or gas-filled eyes, adverse effects were similarly noticed for ICG solutions injected into fluid-filled eyes. In fluid-filled eyes, ICG is further diluted by BSS, thus concentrations of the dye are lower than in air- or gas-filled eyes. Uemura et al. [168] noticed visual field defects in 4 of 7 eyes undergoing ICG-assisted ILM peeling. In this study, 0.6–0.8 ml of ICG at 5.0 mg/ml was injected in the fluid-filled eye (corresponding to concentrations of approximately 0.75–1.0 mg/ml), and left in place for at least 3 min. Predominantly nasal visual field defects were observed when ICG-assisted peeling was performed, while no such damage was seen when ILM peeling was conducted without ICG. Gandorfer et al. [119] reported that 0.2–1.0 ml of ICG at 5.0 mg/ml (corresponding to doses of 1–5 mg) injected into fluid-filled eyes may cause retinal damage even at brief exposure. Assuming a vitreous with a volume of about 4.0 ml, the dose of 1.0–5.0 mg ICG could have resulted in a concentration of 0.25–1.25 mg/ml in this study. The ultrastructural analyses of removed tissues indicated a cleavage plane not at the inner undulating aspect of the ILM, but within innermost retinal layers. No such defects were found when ILM peeling was performed without ICG. The authors concluded

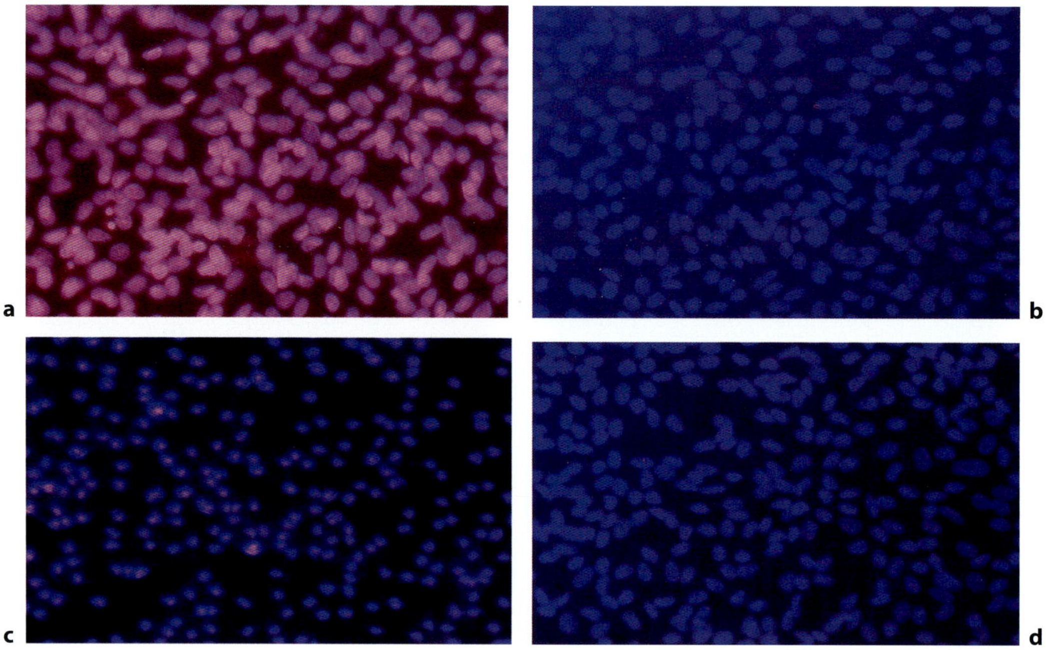

Fig. 3. Photomicrographs displaying cultured human retinal pigment epithelial cells (ARPE-19) stained with DAPI/PI. Blue discloses living cells, red indicates dead cells. **a** Dead cells of the positive control after treatment with 70% ethanol. **b** Living cells after incubation with ICG 5.0 mg/ml for 5 min. **c** Some dead cells after incubation with ICG 5.0 mg/ml under illumination for 5 min. **d** Living cells after incubation with ICG 1.0 mg mg/ml under illumination for 5 min.

that ICG may be responsible for the observed alterations. These observations were partly supported and partly contradicted by several other studies and in vivo and ex vivo studies were performed to investigate this issue.

Nakamura et al. [170] described adverse effects when ILM removal assisted by 0.3 ml of ICG at 5.0 mg/ml (corresponding to a dose of 0.15 mg) was performed in a primate model. The authors found fragments of glial tissues on excised ILM and a damaged vitreoretinal interface, which did not completely recover within 12 months.

Nevertheless, the most relevant data are given by the examination of the excised tissue and the functional outcomes. Kwok et al. [180] using ICG at 0.25 mg/ml also reported adhering cellular elements on the retinal surface of the ILM after ICG-assisted peeling. The morphology of these elements, however, was by far more favorable and the functional results were satisfying. We, like others using low doses and short application time examined our specimens for similar remnants, but could not find cellular elements indicating a disruption plane within the innermost layers (fig. 4). An immunohistological examination with a neuronal marker further excluded a disruption of the neuronal fiber layers (fig. 5).

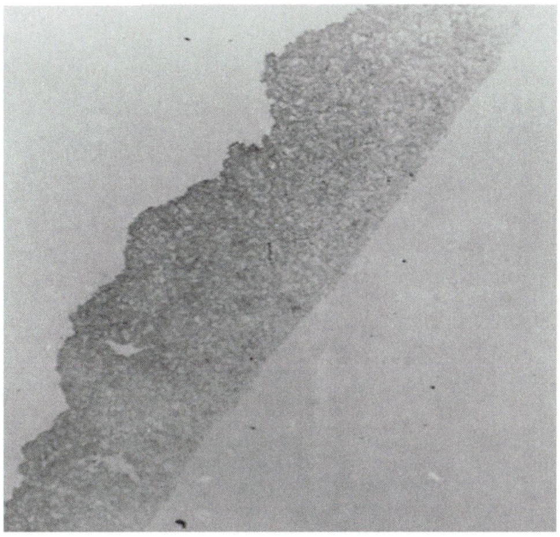

Fig. 4. Electron microscopic view of ILM peeled with ICG (0.25 mg/ml) applied for 15 s. The specimen is completely devoid of cellular remnants.

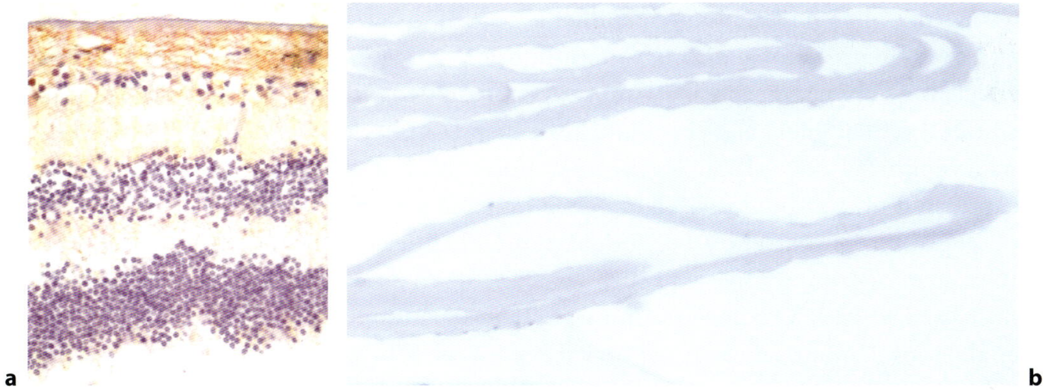

Fig. 5. Photographs displaying a human retina from a donor eye (**a**) and an ILM excised with the help of ICG (0.25 mg/ml) applied for 15 s (**b**). The specimens are probed with an antibody against PGP 9.5. Positive neuronal fibers stained orange-brown can be recognized in the retina but not the ILM.

Taking all contradictory clinical and histological results into account it appears obvious that several factors can influence or enhance negative effects by ICG. These factors can be dissected and analyzed in in vitro experiments. The relevance of the results for clinical practice, however, highly depends on the experimental setup. As an example, Rezai et al. [155] used ICG at 1.0, 5.0 and 20.0 mg/ml and incubated cultured retinal pigment epithelial cells for 30 min with the dye. All concentrations induced a significant amount of apoptosis in retinal pigment epithelial cells already after 24 h of follow-up. Though this study clearly supported the already known information that ICG is not inert, there was no practical relevance with regard to dye concentration and incubation time at all. A clinically more relevant investigation was performed by Ho et al. [165]. The authors incubated cultured retinal pigment epithelial cells with 0.1 ml of ICG at 0.001–5.0 mg/ml (corresponding to doses of 0.0001–0.5 mg) for 5 min up to 3 h. Though concentrations and incubation times partly exceeded clinical practice, the authors made the important observation that cytotoxicity of ICG is dose and time dependent. Morphological changes, as well as reduction of mitochondrial dehydrogenase activity were found for ICG at 5.0 mg/ml after 10 min, at 1.0 mg/ml after 20 min and at 0.01 mg/ml after 3 h. No adverse effects were noticed for the dye-free controls of corresponding osmolarities. The possible mechanism leading to ICG-related toxicity was similarly described by this study group some time later [154, 157]. They considered an Na^+-dependent ICG uptake into retinal pigment epithelial cells responsible for cytotoxicity and increased photosensitizing effects. Removal of sodium in both studies reduced the negative effects of ICG.

Some laboratory studies investigated the effect of different ICG concentrations at exposure times up to 5 min [139, 146, 153], which is closer to clinically relevant dye incubation times. Kodjikian et al. [139] noticed reduced cell viability for ICG at 5.0 mg/ml, when retinal pigment epithelial cell cultures were incubated for 5 min with this dye. No acute toxic effects were found for ICG at 0.5 mg/ml and below. These effects were observed even at a 3-min exposure in two other in vitro studies, one with cultured retinal glial cells [146] and the second similarly with cultured retinal pigment epithelial cells [153]. In the first study, ICG at 5.0 mg/ml caused increased expression of the apoptosis-related gene bcl-2, as well as increased change in morphology in a concentration-dependent manner. Little adverse effects were shown for ICG at 0.5 mg/ml at this exposure time [146]. In the second study, cell viability decreased when ICG concentration was above 0.5 mg/ml [153]. In addition, Tokuda et al. [156] demonstrated retinal toxicity of 0.1 ml ICG at 5.0 mg/ml (corresponding to a dose of 0.5 mg) even at the exposure time of 1 min in an in vitro model with isolated rat retinas. In this study, severe structural damage in every retinal layer and a significantly higher release of lactate dehydrogenase were observed when compared to the use of BSS.

In our study, using the solutions corresponding to doses of 0.5, 0.25 and 0.1 mg, i.e., solutions which mimic the situation in air- or gas-filled eyes, retinal pigment epithelium damage was found only at incubation times beyond 5 min in the setup without illumination. This damage was severe for ICG at 5.0 mg/ml, less severe for ICG at 2.5 mg/ml and little for ICG at 1.0 mg/ml. In this experimental setting, osmolarity of the solutions also seemed to play an important role in observed toxicity while dye-free controls showed similar rates of cell survival and morphologic change. ICG solutions up to a concentration of 0.125 mg/ml, mimicking the situation in fluid-filled eyes, showed no relevant adverse effects in this setup. One reason might be the by far lower dye concentration of the solutions, another that osmolarity was in the physiological range of 295–315 mosm/kg. No changes in cell viability or morphology were observed at all using the solutions at 0.0625 and 0.025 mg/ml, as well as their dye-free controls of corresponding osmolarities. Median cell survival was around 100% and median morphological change never exceeded 1% in every setup conducted.

Recapitulating the results of our study, brief exposure of 1 min or shorter to ICG at 1.0 mg/ml and below seems to cause no acute adverse effects to the retinal pigment epithelium even when illumination is present in clinically relevant limits (<5 min). In contrast, care should be taken using higher-concentrated hypoosmotic ICG solutions of 2.5 mg/ml and more at incubation times beyond 5 min.

Influence of Dye Persistence

Recently, several clinical trials described persistence of ICG in the retina [43, 93, 96, 103, 104, 108, 170] and in other structures of the visual pathway [166, 181]. In these studies, about 0.1–0.3 ml of ICG at 1.25–5.0 mg/ml was applied to the vitreous and left in place for time periods ranging from some seconds to a maximum of 5 min. Both, satisfying visual and functional outcomes as well as severe adverse effects were observed [56, 66, 93].

Weinberger et al. [117] noticed ICG persistence for 6 weeks after macular hole surgery. In their study, a small amount of ICG at 5.0 mg/ml was applied to the vitreous and left in place for 1 min. No evidence for dye-related toxicity could be determined in this study, as well as in a follow-up study with a mean of 8 months conducted by the same group [108]. The authors suggested that the persistent fluorescence signal was due to the low metabolization of ICG in the bradytrophic environment of the remaining adherent vitreous and ILM. Horiguchi et al. [104] similarly reported persisting ICG fluorescence for a mean of 2.7 months after macular hole surgery in 14 patients. In this study, ILM staining was performed with 0.1–0.2 ml of ICG at 1.25 mg/ml, the dye was left in place for approximately 10–30 s and similarly no adverse effects due to ICG were observed. The investigators suggested ICG penetration and/or diffusion into the retina as being responsible for such long dye persistence. Two cases reported by Ashikari et al. [43] showed ICG persistence at the fundus for even longer than 6 months. ICG at 5.0 mg/ml was used, left in place for only a few seconds, and no complications during surgical procedure or complications due to the dye were observed. Ciardella et al. [96], when using ICG at 2.5 mg/ml, demonstrated subfoveal fluorescence persistence up to 8 months after uneventful macular hole surgery in 4 reported cases. The authors' theory was an ICG uptake by the subfoveal retinal pigment epithelium, and this theory was also supported by two studies of Chang et al. [143, 144]. Another clinical investigation by Tadayoni et al. [103] reported, apart from fluorescence persistence, on dye accumulation in the retinal pigment epithelium and the optic nerve. The authors used infracyanine green at a concentration of 2.5 mg/ml and incubated the dye for 3 min. No adverse effects were noticed, but the investigators were concerned about the long-term safety of the dye

[103]. These concerns were consistent with those of Kroemer et al. [181]. This study group worked with almost the same protocol (ICG 2.5 mg/ml for 3 min), and similarly noticed dye accumulation in the area of the former macular hole, retinal axons and around the optic disk. In agreement with previous results, no functional implications and visual field defects were observed in this study.

Da Mata et al. [71] recently published a follow-up study of their original clinical investigation with 114 patients receiving ICG-assisted macular hole surgery. In their original protocol from 1999, 0.2–0.4 ml of ICG at 5.0 mg/ml was used and was left in place for 3–5 min. Shortly thereafter, they showed that adequate ILM staining could also be achieved with 0.05–0.1 ml of ICG at 5.0 mg/ml incubated for 30 s. The study with a mean follow-up of 26 months showed excellent anatomic and visual results, without evidence for dye-related toxicity. To our knowledge, this is the only clinical study with such long follow-up times reporting no adverse effects of ICG. However, these favorable outcomes may be due to the change of the staining technique at an early stage, using lower ICG doses and shorter incubation times.

In contrast to all these studies noticing dye persistence without dye-related toxicity, Cheng et al. [66] showed chronic toxic effects of residual ICG after macular hole surgery in case reports of 6 patients. In this study, 1.0–1.5 ml of ICG at 2.5 mg/ml (corresponding to doses of 2.5–3.75 mg) were instilled in the eyes and left in place for 1–5 min. All eyes had residual ICG left behind at the end of surgery, independent of exposure time. Patients were followed up for 1 year. Circular foveal retinal pigment epithelium atrophy larger than the area of the macular hole and surrounding cuff was noted in 4 of 5 cases with preoperative macular hole. The first retinal damage was already seen 1 month after surgery [19]. These results are certainly concerning, but the used volumes (usually 0.1–0.2 ml) were high and exposure times (usually 10–30 s) long. Closer to the present dye-assisted surgical technique are two other clinical studies reporting on delayed toxicity of ICG [67, 93]. Nakamura et al. [67] reported on ICG persistence for 7.3 months on average and the occurrence of peripheral visual field defects in 2 of 34 eyes which underwent ICG-assisted macular hole surgery. In this study, 0.3 ml of ICG at 5.0 mg/ml (corresponding to a dose of 1.5 mg) was applied to the vitreous and removed immediately by aspiration. In the eyes with visual field defects, ICG persisted at the bottom of the former macular hole and led to retinal pigment epithelial atrophy. These findings match with the case report of Hirata et al. [93], where accidental subretinal migration of ICG leading to retinal pigment epithelium atrophy was described. In the study by Hirata et al. [93], the same volume of solution and the same concentration of ICG were used. Accidental subretinal migration is a dreaded complication during macular hole surgery [182]. During these situations, ICG has direct access to subretinal structures such as the retinal pigment epithelium. Consequently, retinal pigment epithelium damage in the context of ICG persistence demanded further investigation of delayed toxicity of ICG solutions, which has been conducted in numerous experimental studies [139, 153, 161, 162, 164, 171] as well as by our study group.

In our study with cultured ARPE-19 cells, we had follow-up observations at 6, 24 and 72 h after ICG treatment. Although all these above-mentioned clinical trials did not show toxic effects of ICG at the follow-up time of 3 days, there were several animal and in vitro studies reporting negative effects even after some days and even for low-concentrated ICG solutions [159, 171]. Concentration-dependent delayed ICG toxicity was shown by Kawaji et al. [162] in an animal model. These investigators injected 0.05 ml of ICG at concentrations of 25.0, 5.0 and 0.5 mg/ml (corresponding to doses of 1.25, 0.25 and 0.025 mg), as well as BSS into the subretinal space of rabbit eyes. Histological evaluation was performed up to 28 days after injection of ICG at 5.0 mg/ml, as well as at 14 days after injection of the other solutions. Severe retinal pigment epithelium damage was shown for ICG at 25.0 mg/ml after 14 days. In eyes injected with ICG at 5.0 mg/ml the photoreceptors began disappearing within 3 days after the injection and over time developed retinal atrophy. In contrast, no damage to retinal layers was shown for ICG at 0.5 mg/ml and BSS 14 days after injection. Similar results were observed in another animal study by Maia et al. [161], where 0.02 ml of ICG at 5.0 mg/ml (corresponding to a dose of 0.1 mg) was injected into the subretinal space followed by 7 min of endolight illumination at maximum intensity or without light exposure. Animals were followed up for 14 days. First damage to retinal layers was already noticed on the first day after surgery, showing altered photoreceptor segments and degeneration of the outer nuclear layer. Until day 7, light exposure seemed to enforce the damaging potential. On day 14, all retinal layers were severely altered independently of any light exposure. In contrast, no such effects were noticed when 0.3 ml of ICG at 5.0 mg/ml (corresponding to a dose of 1.5 mg) was applied onto the retinal surface, left in place for 1 min and followed by 7 min of illumination. Thus, delayed toxicity of commonly used ICG solutions was demonstrated by both studies. Though minimal remnants may persist after surgery, exposure times of up to 28 days at the described concentrations cannot be compared to the clinical situation and are therefore of limited value. Similarly, Lee at al. [164] found ICG to have toxic effects at concentrations of 1.25 mg/ml or higher when injected into the subretinal space of rabbit eyes. In this study, 0.2–0.3 ml of ICG at up to 5.0 mg/ml (corresponding to doses up to 1.5 mg) was used but removed after 1 min. Eyes were followed up for 4 weeks. After 3 days, significant degenerative changes were found in the retinal pigment epithelial cells, the photoreceptors and the outer nuclear layer when ICG at 1.25 mg/ml (dose 0.25 mg) or higher was injected. Thereafter, the level of cellular damage progressed leading to focal retinal pigment epithelium loss and complete destruction of the outer sensory retina. No significant changes were found for ICG at 0.6 mg/ml (dose 0.12 mg) at all follow-up times.

The results of the aforementioned studies showed that damage to the retinal pigment epithelium was present already in the first 3 days after surgery, when using ICG at 1.25 mg/ml or higher. The results of these studies are in accordance with ours, since prolonged exposure of the dye at certain concentrations clearly induced damage. However, these situations do not mimic clinical practice and can therefore be questioned for their clinical relevance. Nevertheless, an important message that can be derived from these reports is that the dye needs to be removed after application. In our experimental setups mimicking air- or gas-filled eyes, 0.1 ml of ICG at 1.0, 2.5 and 5.0 mg/ml (corresponding to doses of 0.01, 0.25 and 0.5 mg) was applied to the cells. We also noticed delayed damage to our retinal pigment epithelial cell cultures when using similar doses of 0.5 and 0.25 mg ICG. Although the main damage already occurred after 6 h, there was a tendency towards decreasing cell survival and increasing change in morphology with prolongation of the follow-up time in every conducted setup. Additionally to our findings, delayed toxicity of ICG even at lower concentrations has also been reported [151, 171]. Hsu et al. [151] demonstrated in their human retinal pigment epithelial cell culture study that ICG at 0.1 mg/ml still significantly inhibited cell growth at an incubation time of 72 h. Enaida et al. [171] even noticed functional damage to the retina without any apparent morphological change for ICG at 0.025 mg/ml. In their study with rat eyes, 0.05 ml of ICG at 0.025–25.0 mg/ml (corresponding to doses of 0.00125–1.25 mg) was injected into the vitreous. Retinal toxicity was histologically assessed by light microscopy on day 10, and retinal function was evaluated by electroretinography after 10 days, as well as after 2 months. For the higher-concentrated ICG solutions, severe retinal damage with histologically detectable alterations of retinal tissues could be determined. For the lower-concentrated ICG solutions at 0.25 and 0.025 mg/ml, no morphological damage, but decreased amplitudes of dark-adapted a- and b-waves in electroretinograms were detected after 10 days, and there was no recovery within 2 months. However, there are some limitations to these studies, as (a) no irrigation was performed and (b) no clinically relevant incubation times were adhered to.

In contrast to these reports, with ICG solutions at 0.025–0.125 mg/ml (corresponding to doses of 0.0025–0.0125 mg) no chronic toxic effects were found in every setup and at all follow-up times used in our study. To summarize, changes in cell survival and morphology were more prominent for ICG at 1.0 mg/ml and above when comparing the 6-hour time point to the 24-hour time point, than thereafter. This could be explained by the finding that the apoptosis-related gene bax and the cell cycle arrest protein p21 have peak values at 16–24 h after ICG incubation [183]. In conclusion, the results of our study suggest that there is foremost an acute toxic effect of ICG at concentrations above 1.0 mg/ml rather than a chronic toxicity of ICG remnants after dye removal.

Influence of Illumination

Another important criteria in ICG-assisted macular hole surgery is the use of vitrectomy endolights and the possible photosensitizing effects of ICG on retinal tissues. It is well known that the wavelengths emitted by vitrectomy endolights range between 380 and 760 nm [15], and that the absorption maximum of ICG is approximately

700 nm [13–15, 184, 185]. The photosensitizing effects of ICG were described in several ophthalmologic [109, 140, 142, 152, 168, 186] and nonophthalmologic studies [175, 187]. As responsible parameters, dye properties of ICG [13, 14], dye concentration [15, 184, 185], distance of the endolight pipe and duration of light exposure [39, 120], wavelength spectra emitted by vitrectomy endolights [15, 145, 188], as well as the type of the light source [66] were previously reported.

The ICG dye has a complex molecular structure with both hydrophilic and lipophilic properties [13, 14]. Depending on its concentration and the nature of the solvent, ICG tends to form monomers at lower concentrations and aggregates at higher concentrations [185]. Dissolution in physiologic saline solution also favors aggregation, although dissolution to a low concentration may favor monomers [184]. The maximum absorption spectrum is 785 nm for monomers and 690 nm for aggregates [13, 14, 184]. Similar results were noticed recently by Haritoglou et al. [15] in a study investigating light-absorbing properties of different ICG solutions. The authors also found two absorption maxima, one at approximately 700 nm and a second one at 780 nm. Thus, in clinical practice, there is an overlap between the absorption maxima of ICG and the emission curve of the light source (380–760 nm), resulting in a possible photosensitizing effect, especially at higher ICG concentrations. In addition, the effects of short (around 400 nm) as well as of longer wavelengths (beyond 760 nm) in combination with ICG were demonstrated in some studies [109, 186, 190]. As shown in the investigation by Kadonosono et al. [190] for the short wavelengths (400–450 nm) emitted by the light source, the absorption coefficients of ICG were not greater than those of BSS alone, indicating that there is no additional phototoxicity by short-wavelength light using ICG. In contrast, two other studies noticed increased diode laser uptake (absorption maximum at 810 nm) of retinal tissues after ICG-assisted ILM removal in macular hole surgery [109, 186]. The authors concluded that protein binding of residual ICG led to decreased formation of polymers and shifted absorption beyond 785 nm toward a maximum of 810 nm. Similar observations had previously been reported in other studies [13, 14, 184].

Because interaction of ICG and illumination is obvious, numerous experimental studies in this context were conducted, including postmortem studies [160, 163, 169] and cell culture studies [142, 150, 153, 154, 159, 168, 191].

Gandorfer et al. [169] demonstrated in their ex vivo model with 10 human donor eyes (eyes enucleated 16–30 h after death) that exposure of the ICG-stained ILM to wavelengths beyond 620 nm resulted in severe damage to the inner retina, including loss of ILM, cellular disorganization and fragmentation of the cytoplasm. In this study, 0.05 ml of ICG at 0.5 mg/ml (corresponding to a dose of 0.025 mg) was applied for 1 min followed by 3 min of illumination with wavelengths of 380–760 nm. ICG in combination with wavelengths of 380–620 nm disclosed rupture of Müller cells with detachment of the ILM, but no other cellular disorganization. Eyes subjected to illumination only showed no such abnormalities. These results are consistent with findings of Haritoglou et al. [160] using ICG at 0.5 mg/ml diluted with glucose 5% in combination with endolight illumination (380–760 nm) in a postmortem study 1 year later. The investigators reported disorganization of the inner retina and complete loss of ILM after application of the dye and illumination. No abnormalities were found without illumination and in unstained control specimens. Contrary to these outcomes, in our postmortem study with porcine eyes (eyes processed within 5 h after death) and similar experiments no alteration of retinal structures was detected even at higher ICG concentrations [163]. In this study, 0.5 ml of ICG at 0.1–2.0 mg/ml (corresponding to doses of 0.05–1.0 mg) was applied and left in place for either 30 or 60 s. After irrigation, the posterior pole was irradiated at maximum power for 3 min by a standard light pipe. Although differences between the species may contribute to these contradictory results, according to the authors it was conceivable that the postmortem time and the vitality of the tissue influenced the outcome in this ex vivo system. In fact, Wolf et al. [99] repeated the experiment closely mimicking the clinical situation on an eye shortly after the donor died. This study on a human eye showed similar favorable outcomes as the study with porcine tissue [163].

In numerous cell culture studies testing the effects of ICG with illumination, mainly performed with cultured retinal pigment epithelial cells, phototoxic effects have been noticed [142, 154, 159, 168, 191].

Sippy et al. [191] reported about negative effects of ICG treatment combined with illumination. In this study, cultured human retinal pigment epithelial cells were exposed for 20 min to ICG at 1.0 mg/ml followed by 10 min of endolight illumination. One observed effect was decreased mitochondrial enzyme activity, compared to cells exposed only to BSS and illumination. Paradoxically, no alterations of cellular morphology or ultrastructure were seen. In the study by Ho et al. [154], cultured retinal pigment epithelial cells were exposed to ICG at 2.5 mg/ml either dissolved in BSS or in sodium-free BSS for 2 min. Afterwards, the cells were irradiated with a light beam for 40 min. The authors found photoreactive changes in retinal pigment epithelial cells. These changes included cell shrinkage, cell death, pyknotic nuclei, reduced viability as well as reduced mitochondrial dehydrogenase activity. These effects were less severe when ICG was dissolved in sodium-free BSS. In another study by the same group, Na^+-dependent ICG uptake in retinal pigment epithelial cells was reported to be responsible for such observations [154]. In the same context of photoreactive changes in the retinal pigment epithelium, Yam et al. [168] reported concentration-dependent toxicity of ICG solutions in combination with acute endolight illumination on cultured retinal pigment epithelial cells. In this study, ICG at 0.25 and 2.5 mg/ml was applied to cultured ARPE-19 cells for 1 min. After isotonic rinsing, the cells were irradiated with a light beam (400–800 nm) at a distance of 10 mm for 15 min. Cell viability decreased to 40% for ICG at 2.5 mg/ml and to 80% for ICG at 0.25 mg/ml, respectively. The authors similarly noticed an upregulation of the apoptosis-related genes p63 and bax, as well as the gene for the cell cycle arrest protein p21. Contrary to these findings, Iriyama et al. [159] noticed no affection of cell viability of cultured retinal glial cells when using a similar protocol. This aspect is remarkable, while another in vitro study using both cell lines suggested cultured retinal pigment epithelial cells to be more resistant to light exposure after brief incubation with ICG than cultured retinal glial cells [150]. The different sensitivity of retinal cells was similarly shown by the study of Narayanan et al. [142], comparing ICG effects accompanied by 10 min of illumination on viability of cultured human retinal pigment epithelial cells and rat neurosensory retinal cells (R28). In this study, ICG caused a significant decrease in mitochondrial dehydrogenase activity in R28 and ARPE-19 cells. ICG without light exposure did not decrease mitochondrial dehydrogenase activity. In both cell lines, [^{3}H]thymidine incorporation was increased when treated with ICG with or without light indicating increased DNA synthesis. Surprisingly, R28 cells did not show any significant decrease in cell viability. Closer to clinically relevant illumination times, Gale et al. [153] tested the effects of 0.75 ml ICG at 0.5 and 2.5 mg/ml (corresponding to doses of 0.375 and 1.875 mg) in combination with illumination on cultured retinal pigment epithelial cells. Each solution was applied to the cells for 5 min coupled with 1 min of intense fiber-optic illumination. Although there was a reduction of cell viability for both dyes, no significant differences were noticed when results were compared to those without the use of illumination. Therefore, according to this study, there seems to be a toxic effect of ICG independent of additional light exposure.

Regarding these contradictory clinical and experimental results, we decided to test the effects of ICG combined with illumination on the retinal pigment epithelium in our in vitro study. In the setup with illumination, cultured ARPE-19 cells were exposed to ICG at 0.025–5.0 mg/ml for either 1 or 5 min coupled with illumination by a standard halogen vitrectomy endolight pipe (380–760 nm) at a distance of 8 mm [163, 169]. Phototoxicity was not present with the dye-free controls of corresponding osmolarities, as well as with the diluted ICG solutions at 0.125 mg/ml and below used to mimic the situation that occurs in fluid-filled eyes. Severely decreased cell viability and an increase in morphological change were found for ICG at 5.0 mg/ml at both incubation and illumination times. After the follow-up time of 72 h, we noticed median cell survival of 85% after 1 and 66% after 5 min of incubation and illumination as well as median morphologic change of 15% after 1 and 41% after 5 min. Similarly, with growing incubation and illumination times, median cell survival was decreased and median morphological change was increased to a lesser degree for ICG at 2.5 mg/ml (cell survival >89%, morphologic change <12%) and to a small degree for ICG at 1.0 mg/ml (cell survival >98%, morphologic change <3%).

To summarize, phototoxicity of ICG is concentration and illumination time dependent, when ICG is used at concentrations above 1.0 mg/ml, mimicking air- or gas-filled eyes at illumination times up to 5 min. ICG below 1.0 mg/ml coupled with illumination of 1 min or shorter appears to be safe in our in vitro model. Concerning the type of illumination used during ICG-assisted macular hole surgery, one study with postmortem eyes showed more favorable outcomes for the xenon light source compared to the halogen light source [145].

Influence of Osmolarity

The influence of hypoosmotic solvent solutions for ICG is a controversially discussed topic when using ICG preparations [15, 153, 192]. ICG powder is primarily not soluble in BSS, but only in distilled aqueous solution (ICG solvent) at very low osmolarity. Thus, ICG solutions frequently used in macular hole surgery for air- or gas-filled eyes, ICG 1.0–5.0 mg/ml, are often hypoosmotic. No such problems occur if ICG is further diluted by BSS when applied to fluid-filled eyes. Osmolarity of these ICG dyes are within physiological limits (295–315 mosm/kg). Furthermore, it is important to notice that there is still no standardized dilution protocol for ICG solutions and that there are remarkable differences in osmolarity of similar-concentrated ICG solutions depending on the proportions of solvent solution and BSS in the final ICG preparation. For example, the osmolarity of ICG at 1.0 mg/ml ranged from around 240 [153] to 299 mosm/kg [154] in different investigations. Stalmans et al. [192] demonstrated adverse effects of hypoosmotic ICG and solvent solutions in a study with retinal pigment epithelial cells. The outcomes of cell survival using ICG at 1.0 mg/ml of 248 mosm/kg as well as the dye-free control solution of 247 mosm/kg were compared to outcomes when using BSS (311 mosm/kg) and other isoosmotic solutions. The investigators noticed a significantly decreased cell viability for ICG and its dye-free control solution compared to the other solutions after an exposure time of 5 min. No statistically significant difference was found comparing these two hypoosmotic solutions ($p = 0.78$). In contrast to these findings, Gale et al. [153] reported significant differences in the outcomes of cell survival, when the hypoosmotic ICG at 1.0 mg/ml (240 mosm/kg) was compared to the similarly hypoosmotic dye-free control (242 mosm/kg) at an incubation time of 3 min. They reported 103.7% cell survival for the dye-free solution compared to 89.9% for ICG at 1.0 mg/ml. These differences became even more prominent when ICG at 2.5 and 5.0 mg/ml were compared to their dye-free controls.

In our study, osmolarities were 290, 277 and 242 mosm/kg for ICG at 1.0, 2.5 and 5.0 mg/ml, respectively. For the diluted ICG at 0.025, 0.0625 and 0.125 mg/ml, we measured 307, 303 and 297 mosm/kg, respectively. To test the effects of osmolarity without interfering parameters such as illumination, we performed our in vitro experiments with ICG solutions and BSS/solvent mixes of corresponding osmolarities at incubation times up to 20 min in the dark. Although we noticed statistically significant differences in cell survival ($p = 0.0057$) and morphologic change ($p = 0.0014$) depending on whether or not the solutions contained ICG, the differences between the outcomes were small and not clinically relevant. Median cell survival for ICG at 5.0 mg/ml, after the follow-up time of 72 h, was 93% after 5, 18% after 10 and even 0% after 20 min of incubation time. For the dye-free control, after the same follow-up time, it was 93% after 5, 22% after 10 and 0% after 20 min. The differences became even smaller when outcomes of ICG at 2.5 and 1.0 mg/ml were compared to their dye-free controls. As expected, there were no adverse effects for

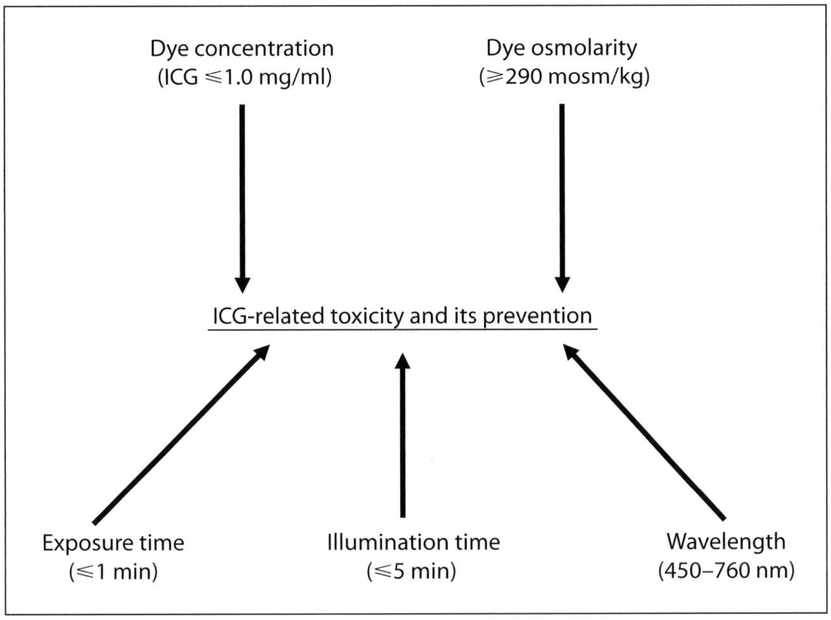

Fig. 6. Aspects leading to dye-related toxicity and its prevention in vitreoretinal surgery.

isoosmotic ICG solutions in our study, even after the maximum incubation time of 20 min.

To summarize, there is obviously an effect of osmolarity in higher-concentrated ICG solutions on survival and morphology of cultured retinal pigment epithelial cells. Isoosmotic ICG solutions below 1.0 mg/ml appeared to be safe at incubation times up to 20 min without the use of illumination. Hypoosmotic ICG solutions, as used in air- or gas-filled eyes, only seemed to be safe when incubation times were kept below 5 min and no illumination was used.

Summary and Conclusions

ICG can without doubt exert cytotoxic effects. On the other hand, it is still a useful dye for macular hole surgery in combination with ILM peeling. Therefore, surgeons working with this vital stain should note the following aspects for a safe accomplishment of ILM peeling or ERM removal (fig. 6).

The toxic effects of ICG on the retinal pigment epithelium are widespread and complex. The results of several studies as well as our experimental workup showed that ICG toxicity to the retinal pigment epithelium is dependent on the dye concentration, the osmolarity of the solvent solutions, as well as on the lengths of dye exposure time and vitrectomy endolight illumination time. For this reason, we recommend the use of isoosmolar ICG solutions (osmolarity ≥290 mosm/kg) with a concentration of 1.0 mg/ml or less. In addition, we recommend to keep the exposure and the illumination times as short as possible, and to make sure that the dye is removed as thoroughly as possible by irrigation or aspiration. An incubation time of 1 min, which is twice or thrice the time nowadays applied, followed by an illumination time of 5 min or less appeared to be safe in our in vitro study, when ICG at concentrations of 1.0 mg/ml or less was used.

To summarize, there is still no standardized protocol for ICG-assisted ILM or ERM staining during macular hole surgery, and the parameters responsible for ICG-induced toxicity are still controversial. Thus, further investigations which consider most of the parameters that occur in clinical practice (appropriate dye concentrations and exposure times as well as vitrectomy endolight illumination) are required.

In recent as well as in past clinical and experimental studies, several publications addressed both positive and negative effects of vital stains. It is indisputable that the introduction and use of ICG and other dyes for ILM peeling and ERM removal in vitreoretinal surgery facilitated the work of numerous surgeons. The introduction of ICG into vitreoretinal surgery clearly lacked sufficient safety data and many negative experiences might have been avoided if the chronology of experimental and clinical use had not been inverted. Nevertheless, this experience was a good lesson, and novel but not completely inert vital dyes are explored more carefully now before being introduced in clinics.

References

1 Kelly NE, Wendel RT: Vitreous surgery for idiopathic macular holes. Results of a pilot study. Arch Ophthalmol 1991;109:654–659.
2 Ezra E, Aylward WG, Gregor ZJ: Membranectomy and autologous serum for the retreatment of full-thickness macular holes. Arch Ophthalmol 1997; 115:1276–1280.
3 Liggett PE, Skolik DS, Horio B, Saito Y, Alfaro V, Mieler W: Human autologous serum for the treatment of full-thickness macular holes. A preliminary study. Ophthalmology 1995;102:1071–1076.
4 Olsen TW, Sternberg P Jr, Capone A Jr, Martin DF, Lim JI, Grossniklaus HE, Aaberg TM Sr: Macular hole surgery using thrombin-activated fibrinogen and selective removal of the internal limiting membrane. Retina 1998;18:322–329.
5 Tornambe PE, Poliner LS, Grote K: Macular hole surgery without face-down positioning. A pilot study. Retina 1997;17:179–185.
6 Brooks HL Jr: Macular hole surgery with and without internal limiting membrane peeling. Ophthalmology 2000;107:1939–1948.
7 Mester V, Kuhn F: Internal limiting membrane removal in the management of full-thickness macular holes. Am J Ophthalmol 2000;129:769–777.
8 Krovetz LJ, Gessner IH: A new method utilizing indicator-dilution techniques for estimation of left-to-right shunts in infants. Circulation 1965;32: 772–777.
9 Winkler K, Larsen JA, Munker T, Tygstrup N: Determination of the hepatic blood flow in man by simultaneous use of five test substances measured in two parts of the liver. Scand J Clin Lab Invest 1965; 17:423–432.
10 Leevy CM, Smith F, Longueville J, Paumgartner G, Howard MM: Indocyanine green clearance as a test for hepatic function. Evaluation by dichromatic ear densitometry. JAMA 1967;200:236–240.
11 Flower RW: Injection technique for indocyanine green and sodium fluorescein dye angiography of the eye. Invest Ophthalmol 1973;12:881–895.
12 McEnerney JK, Peyman GA: Indocyanine green: a new vital stain for use before penetrating keratoplasty. Arch Ophthalmol 1978;96:1445–1447.

13 Mordon S, Devoisselle JM, Soulie-Begu S, Desmettre T: Indocyanine green: physicochemical factors affecting its fluorescence in vivo. Microvasc Res 1998; 55:146–152.
14 Desmettre T, Devoisselle JM, Mordon S: Fluorescence properties and metabolic features of indocyanine green (ICG) as related to angiography. Surv Ophthalmol 2000;45:15–27.
15 Haritoglou C, Gandorfer A, Schaumberger M, Tadayoni R, Kampik A: Light-absorbing properties and osmolarity of indocyanine-green depending on concentration and solvent medium. Invest Ophthalmol Vis Sci 2003;44:2722–2729.
16 Garski TR, Staller BJ, Hepner G, Banka VS, Finney RA Jr: Adverse reactions after administration of indocyanine green. JAMA 1978;240:635.
17 Benya R, Quintana J, Brundage B: Adverse reactions to indocyanine green: a case report and a review of the literature. Cathet Cardiovasc Diagn 1989;17: 231–233.
18 Hoppe-Ross M: Adverse reactions due to indocyanine green. Ophthalmology 1994;101:529–533.
19 Yannuzzi LA, Slakter JS, Sorenson JA, Guyer DR, Orlock DA: Digital indocyanine green videoangiography and choroidal neovascularization. Retina 1992; 12:191–223.
20 Horiguchi M: Staining of the lens capsule for circular continuous capsulorrhexis in eyes with white cataract. Arch Ophthalmol 1998;116:535–537.
21 Kadonosono K, Itoh N, Uchio E, Nakamura S, Ohno S: Staining of internal limiting membrane in macular hole surgery. Arch Ophthalmol 2000;118: 1116–1118.
22 Kusaka S, Nobutsugu H, Ohji M, Hayashi A, Kamei M, Tano Y: Indocyanine green facilitates removal of epiretinal and internal limiting membranes in myopic eyes with retinal detachment. Am J Ophthalmol 2001; 131:388–390.
23 Grizzard WS, Tornambe PE: Indocyanine green used as a vital dye to assist in the identification and removal of surface retinal membranes (abstract). Proc 22nd Meeting Club Jules Gonin, 2000, p 133.
24 Querques G, Prascina F, Iaculli C, Noci ND: Retinal toxicity of indocyanine green. Int Ophthalmol, E-pub ahead of print.
25 Arevalo JF, Garcia RA: Macular hole surgery complicated by accidental massive subretinal indocyanine green, and retinal tear. Graefes Arch Clin Exp Ophthalmol 2007;245:751–753.
26 Sayanagi K, Ikuno Y, Soga K, Sawa M, Oshima Y, Kamei M, Kusaka S, Tano Y: Residual indocyanine green fluorescence pattern after vitrectomy for idiopathic macular hole with internal limiting membrane peeling. Br J Ophthalmol 2007;91:939–944.
27 Hillenkamp J, Saikia P, Herrmann WA, Framme C, Gabel VP, Sachs HG: Surgical removal of idiopathic epiretinal membrane with or without the assistance of indocyanine green: a randomised controlled clinical trial. Graefes Arch Clin Exp Ophthalmol 2007; 245:973–979.
28 Lai MM, Williams GA: Anatomical and visual outcomes of idiopathic macular hole surgery with internal limiting membrane removal using low-concentration indocyanine green. Retina 2007;27: 477–482.
29 Tsuiki E, Fujikawa A, Miyamura N, Yamada K, Mishima K, Kitaoka T: Visual field defects after macular hole surgery with indocyanine green-assisted internal limiting membrane peeling. Am J Ophthalmol 2007;143:704–705.
30 Beutel J, Dahmen G, Ziegler A, Hoerauf H: Internal limiting membrane peeling with indocyanine green or trypan blue in macular hole surgery: a randomized trial. Arch Ophthalmol 2007;125:326–332.
31 Sekiryu T, Iida T: Long-term observation of fundus infrared fluorescence after indocyanine green-assisted vitrectomy. Retina 2007;27:190–197.
32 Oie Y, Emi K, Takaoka G, Ikeda T: Effect of indocyanine green staining in peeling of internal limiting membrane for retinal detachment resulting from macular hole in myopic eyes. Ophthalmology 2007;114:303–306.
33 Ullern M, Dubreuil F, Nourry H, Poisson F, Baudouin C: Macular hole surgery with and without infracyanine-green-guided removal of the internal limiting membrane. J Fr Ophthalmol 2007;30:53–57.
34 Lai TY, Kwok AK, Au AW, Lam DS: Assessment of macular function by multifocal electroretinography following epiretinal membrane surgery with indocyanine green-assisted internal limiting membrane peeling. Graefes Arch Clin Exp Ophthalmol 2007; 245:148–154.
35 Rufer F, Frimpong-Boateng A, Bunse A, Roider J: Comparison of ILM peeling with and without the use of indocyanine green. Functional results for idiopathic macular hole after pars plana vitrectomy. Ophthalmologe 2007;104:54–59.
36 Bardak Y, Cekic O, Tig SU: Comparison of ICG-assisted ILM peeling and triamcinolone-assisted posterior vitreous removal in diffuse diabetic macular oedema. Eye 2006;20:1357–1359.
37 Saito M, Iida T: A surgical technique to protect the macular hole in indocyanine green-assisted vitrectomy. Ophthalmic Surg Lasers Imaging 2006;37: 511–515.
38 Ferencz M, Somfai GM, Farkas A, Kovacs I, Lesch B, Recsan Z, Nemes J, Salacz G: Functional assessment of the possible toxicity of indocyanine green dye in macular hole surgery. Am J Ophthalmol 2006;142:765–770.

39 Schaal KB, Bartz-Schmidt KU, Dithmar S: Current strategies for macular hole surgery in Germany, Austria and Switzerland. Ophthalmologe 2006;103: 922–926.
40 Wrede J, Engler C, Dithmar S: Functional results after anatomically successful surgery for stage III/IV macular hole. Ophthalmologe 2006;103:935–939.
41 Villota-Deleu E, Castro-Navarro J, Gonzalez-Castano C, Perez-Carro G: Outcomes of macular hole surgery using three different surgical techniques. Arch Soc Esp Oftalmol 2006;81:581–590.
42 Ueno S, Kondo M, Piao CH, Ikenoya K, Miyake Y, Terasaki H: Selective amplitude reduction of the PhNR after macular hole surgery: ganglion cell damage related to ICG-assisted ILM peeling and gas tamponade. Invest Ophthalmol Vis Sci 2006;47: 3545–3549.
43 Ashikari M, Ozeki H, Tomida K, Sakurai E, Tamai K, Ogura Y: Long-term retention of dye after indocyanine green-assisted internal limiting membrane peeling. Jpn J Ophthalmol 2006;50:349–353.
44 Kumagai K, Furukawa M, Ogino N, Uemura A, Larson E: Long-term outcomes of internal limiting membrane peeling with and without indocyanine green in macular hole surgery. Retina 2006;26: 613–617.
45 Rizzo S, Belting C, Genovesi-Ebert F, Vento A, Cresti F: Modified technique for safer indocyanine-green-assisted peeling of the internal limiting membrane during vitrectomy for macular hole repair. Graefes Arch Clin Exp Ophthalmol 2006;244:1615–1619.
46 Husson-Danan A, Glacet-Bernard A, Soubrane G, Coscas G: Clinical evaluation of the use of indocyanine green for peeling the internal limiting membrane in macular hole surgery. Graefes Arch Clin Exp Ophthalmol 2006;244:291–297.
47 Allen RC, Russell SR, Schluter ML, Oetting TA: Retained posterior segment indocyanine green dye after phacoemulsification. J Cataract Refract Surg 2006;32:357–360.
48 Mavrofrides E, Smiddy WE, Kitchens JW, Salicone A, Feuer W: Indocyanine green-assisted internal limiting membrane peeling for macular holes: toxicity? Retina 2006;26:637–644.
49 Shah SP, Patel M, Thomas D, Aldington S, Laidlaw DA: Factors predicting outcome of vitrectomy for diabetic macular oedema: results of a prospective study. Br J Ophthalmol 2006;90:33–36.
50 La Heij EC, Dieudonne SC, Mooy CM, Diederen RM, Liem AT, van Suylen RJ, Hendrikse F: Immunohistochemical analysis of the internal limiting membrane peeled with infracyanine green. Am J Ophthalmol 2005;140:1123–1125.
51 Koestinger A, Bovey EH: Visual acuity after vitrectomy and epiretinal membrane peeling with or without premacular indocyanine green injection. Eur J Ophthalmol 2005;15:795–799.
52 Oficjalska-Mlynczak J, Jamrozy-Witkowska A, Muzyka-Wozniak M, Krzyzanowska P: Outcome results in macular hole surgery with internal limiting membrane removal. Klin Oczna 2005;107: 650–653.
53 Hager A, Ehrich S, Wiegand W: Anatomical and functional results after elective macular surgery. Ophthalmologe 2005;102:597–602.
54 Uemoto R, Yamamoto S, Takeuchi S: Changes in retinal pigment epithelium after indocyanine green-assisted internal limiting lamina peeling during macular hole surgery. Am J Ophthalmol 2005;140: 752–755.
55 Kersey TL, Bolton A, Patel CK: Serial autofluorescence imaging over two years following indocyanine green-assisted internal limiting membrane peel for macular hole. Clin Exp Ophthalmol 2005; 33:538–539.
56 Nakamura H, Hayakawa K, Sawaguchi S, Gaja T: Removal of retinal indocyanine green dye by autologous serum irrigation in macular hole surgery. Retina 2005;25:736–741.
57 Lai CC, Wu WC, Chuang LH, Yeung L, Lee JS, Chen TL: Selective staining of the internal limiting membrane using the sequential intraoperative instillation of whole blood followed by indocyanine green dye. Am J Ophthalmol 2005;140:320–322.
58 Lai CC, Wu WC, Chuang LH, Yeung L, Chen TL, Lin KK: Prevention of indocyanine green toxicity on retinal pigment epithelium with whole blood in stain-assisted macular hole surgery. Ophthalmology 2005;112:1409–1414.
59 Jaycock PD, Bunce C, Xing W, Thomas D, Poon W, Gazzard G, Williamson TH, Laidlaw DA: Outcomes of macular hole surgery: implications for surgical management and clinical governance. Eye 2005;19: 879–884.
60 Kamura Y, Sato Y, Isomae T, Shimada H: Effects of internal limiting membrane peeling in vitrectomy on diabetic cystoid macular edema patients. Jpn J Ophthalmol 2005;49:297–300.
61 Lee KL, Dean S, Guest S: A comparison of outcomes after indocyanine green and trypan blue assisted internal limiting membrane peeling during macular hole surgery. Br J Ophthalmol 2005;89:420–424.
62 Hillenkamp J, Saikia P, Gora F, Sachs HG, Lohmann CP, Roider J, Baumler W, Gabel VP: Macular function and morphology after peeling of idiopathic epiretinal membrane with and without the assistance of indocyanine green. Br J Ophthalmol 2005; 89:437–443.
63 Tognetto D, Haritoglou C, Kampik A, Ravalico G: Macular edema and visual loss after macular pucker surgery with ICG-assisted internal limiting membrane peeling. Eur J Ophthalmol 2005;15:289–291.

64 Wang HH, Wu TT, Sheu SJ: Treatment of macular holes with indocyanine green-assisted retinal internal limiting membrane peeling. Kaohsiung J Med Sci 2005;21:108–113.

65 Posselt D, Rahman R, Smith M, Simcock PR: Visual outcomes following ICG assisted ILM peel for macular hole. Eye 2005;19:279–283.

66 Cheng SN, Yang TC, Ho JD, Hwang JF, Cheng CK: Ocular toxicity of intravitreal indocyanine green. J Ocul Pharmacol Ther 2005;21:85–93.

67 Nakamura H, Hayakawa K, Imaizumi A, Sakai M, Sawaguchi S: Persistence of retinal indocyanine green dye following vitreous surgery. Ophthalmic Surg Lasers Imaging 2005;36:37–45.

68 Sakaguchi H, Ikuno Y, Choi JS, Ohji M, Tano T: Multiple components of epiretinal tissues detected by triamcinolone and indocyanine green in macular hole and retinal detachment as a result of high myopia. Am J Ophthalmol 2004;138:1079–1081.

69 Ando F, Yasui O, Hirose H, Ohba N: Optic nerve atrophy after vitrectomy with indocyanine green-assisted internal limiting membrane peeling in diffuse diabetic macular edema. Adverse effect of ICG-assisted ILM peeling. Graefes Arch Clin Exp Ophthalmol 2004;242:995–999.

70 Ando F, Sasano K, Suzuki F, Ohba N: Indocyanine green-assisted ILM peeling in macular hole surgery revisited. Am J Ophthalmol 2004;138:886–887.

71 Da Mata AP, Burk SE, Foster RE, Riemann CD, Petersen MR, Nehemy MB, Augsburger JJ: Long-term follow-up of indocyanine green-assisted peeling of the retinal internal limiting membrane during vitrectomy surgery for idiopathic macular hole repair. Ophthalmology 2004;11:2246–2253.

72 Brazitikos PD, Androudi S, Tsinopoulos I, Papadopoulos NT, Balidis M, Georgiadis N: Functional and anatomic results of macular hole surgery complicated by massive indocyanine green subretinal migration. Acta Ophthalmol Scand 2004;2:613–515.

73 Kanda S, Uemura A, Yamashita T, Kita H, Yamakiri K, Sakamoto T: Visual field defects after intravitreous administration of indocyanine green in macular hole surgery. Arch Ophthalmol 2004;122:1447–1451.

74 Avci R, Kaderli B, Avci B, Simsek S, Baykara M, Kahveci Z, Gelisken O, Yucel AA: Pars plana vitrectomy and removal of the internal limiting membrane in the treatment of chronic macular oedema. Graefes Arch Clin Exp Ophthalmol 2004;242: 845–852.

75 Kwok AK, Lai TY, Li WW, Yew DT, Wong VW: Trypan blue- and indocyanine green-assisted epiretinal membrane surgery: clinical and histopathological studies. Eye 2004;18:882–888.

76 Kwok AK, Lai TY, Li WW, Woo DC, Chan NR: Indocyanine green-assisted internal limiting membrane removal in epiretinal membrane surgery: a clinical and histologic study. Am J Ophthalmol 2004; 138:194–199.

77 Lochhead J, Jones E, Chui D, Lake S, Karia N, Patel CK, Rosen P: Outcome of ICG-assisted ILM peel in macular hole surgery. Eye 2004;18:804–808.

78 Avci R, Avci B, Kaderli B, Cavusoglu I: A new surgical approach for indocyanine green-assisted internal limiting membrane peeling. Ophthalmic Surg Lasers Imaging 2004;35:292–297.

79 Horio N, Horiguchi M: Effect on visual outcome after macular hole surgery when staining the internal limiting membrane with indocyanine green dye. Arch Ophthalmol 2004;122:992–996.

80 Hirata A, Tanihara H: Ruptured internal limiting membrane associated with blunt trauma revealed by indocyanine green staining. Graefes Arch Clin Exp Ophthalmol 2004;242:527–530.

81 Kromer I, Lommatzsch A, Pauleikhoff D: Retinal ICG-accumulation after ILM-staining during macular hole surgery? Ophthalmologe 2004;101:604–607.

82 Facino M, Mochi B, Lai S, Terrile R: A simple way to prevent indocyanine green from entering the subretinal space during vitrectomy for retinal detachment due to myopic macular hole. Eur J Ophthalmol 2004; 14:269–271.

83 Schmidt JC, Rodrigues EB, Meyer CH, Hoerle S, Kroll P: A modified technique to stain the internal limiting membrane with indocyanine green. Ophthalmologica 2004;218:176–179.

84 Radetzky S, Walter P, Fauser S, Koizumi K, Kirchhof B, Joussen AM: Visual outcome of patients with macular edema after pars plana vitrectomy and indocyanine green-assisted peeling of the internal limiting membrane. Graefes Arch Clin Exp Ophthalmol 2004; 242:273–278.

85 Rezende FA, Kapusta MA: Internal limiting membrane: ultrastructural relationships, with clinical implications for macular hole healing. Can J Ophthalmol 2004;39:251–259.

86 Slaughter K, Lee IL: Macular hole surgery with and without indocyanine green assistance. Eye 2004;18: 376–378.

87 Ben Simon GJ, Desatnik H, Alhalel A, Treister G, Moisseiev J: Retrospective analysis of vitrectomy with and without internal limiting membrane peeling for stage 3 and 4 macular hole. Ophthalmic Surg Lasers Imaging 2004;35:109–115.

88 Kuo HK, Lin JW, Kao ML, Liu CC: Clinicopathological study of the idiopathic macular hole: comparison of epiretinal membrane peeling and internal limiting membrane peeling. Ophthalmologica 2004; 218:31–35.

89 Kwok AK, Lai TY, Yuen KS, Tam BS, Wong VW: Macular hole surgery with or without indocyanine green stained internal limiting membrane peeling. Clin Exp Ophthalmol 2003;31:470–475.
90 Sheidow TG, Blinder KJ, Holekamp N, Joseph D, Shah G, Grand MG, Thomas MA, Bakal J, Sharma S: Outcome results in macular hole surgery: an evaluation of internal limiting membrane peeling with and without indocyanine green. Ophthalmology 2003; 110:1697–1701.
91 Gass CA, Haritoglou C, Schaumberger M, Kampik A: Functional outcome of macular hole surgery with and without indocyanine green-assisted peeling of the internal limiting membrane. Graefes Arch Clin Exp Ophthalmol 2003;241:716–720.
92 Haritoglou C, Neubauer AS, Gandorfer A, Thiel M, Kampik A: Indocyanine green for successful repair of a long-standing macular hole. Am J Ophthalmol 2003;136:389–391.
93 Hirata A, Inomata Y, Kawaji T, Tanihara H: Persistent subretinal indocyanine green induces retinal pigment epithelium atrophy. Am J Ophthalmol 2003; 136:353–355.
94 Uemura A, Kanda S, Sakamoto Y, Kita H: Visual field defects after uneventful vitrectomy for epiretinal membrane with indocyanine green-assisted internal limiting membrane peeling. Am J Ophthalmol 2003; 136:252–257.
95 Kwok AK, Lai TY, Yew DT, Li WW: Internal limiting membrane staining with various concentrations of indocyanine green dye under air in macular surgeries. Am J Ophthalmol 2003;136:223–230.
96 Ciardella AP, Schiff W, Barile G, Vidne O, Sparrow J, Langton K, Chang S: Persistent indocyanine green fluorescence after vitrectomy for macular hole. Am J Ophthalmol 2003;136:174–177.
97 Ashikari M, Ozeki H, Tomida K, Sakurai E, Tamai K, Ogura Y: Retention of dye after indocyanine green-assisted internal limiting membrane peeling. Am J Ophthalmol 2003;136:172–174.
98 Kwok AK, Lai TY: Internal limiting membrane removal in macular hole surgery for severely myopic eyes: a case-control study. Br J Ophthalmol 2003;87:885–889.
99 Wolf S, Reichel MB, Wiedemann P, Schnurrbusch UE: Clinical findings in macular hole surgery with indocyanine green-assisted peeling of the internal limiting membrane. Graefes Arch Clin Exp Ophthalmol 2003;241:589–592.
100 Sorcinelli R: Surgical management of epiretinal membrane with indocyanine-green-assisted peeling. Ophthalmologica 2003;217:107–110.
101 Haritoglou C, Gandorfer A, Gass CA, Schaumberger M, Ulbig MW, Kampik A: The effect of indocyanine-green on functional outcome of macular pucker surgery. Am J Ophthalmol 2003;135:328–337.
102 Castro Navarro J, Gonzalez-Castano C: Macular hole surgery with and without internal limiting membrane peeling. Arch Soc Esp Oftalmol 2003;78:159–164.
103 Tadayoni R, Paques M, Girmens JF, Massin P, Gaudric A: Persistence of fundus fluorescence after use of indocyanine green for macular surgery. Ophthalmology 2003;110:604–608.
104 Horiguchi M, Nagata S, Yamamoto N, Kojima Y, Shimada Y: Kinetics of indocyanine green dye after intraocular surgeries using indocyanine green staining. Arch Ophthalmol 2003;121:327–331.
105 Kwok AK, Lai TY, Man-Chan W, Woo DC: Indocyanine green assisted retinal internal limiting membrane removal in stage 3 or 4 macular hole surgery. Br J Ophthalmol 2003;87:71–74.
106 Kube T, Hermel M, Dahlke C, Hutschenreuter G, Schrage N, Kirchhof B: Macular hole surgery: experience with autologous platelet concentrate and indocyanine green-assisted internal limiting membrane peeling. Klin Monatsbl Augenheilkd 2002; 219:883–888.
107 Haritoglou C, Gandorfer A, Gass CA, Schaumberger M, Ulbig MW, Kampik A: Indocyanine green-assisted peeling of the internal limiting membrane in macular hole surgery affects visual outcome: a clinicopathologic correlation. Am J Ophthalmol 2002; 134:836–841.
108 Weinberger AW, Schlossmacher B, Dahlke C, Hermel M, Kirchhof B, Schrage NF: Indocyanine-green-assisted internal limiting membrane peeling in macular hole surgery – A follow-up study. Graefes Arch Clin Exp Ophthalmol 2002;240:913–917.
109 Blem RI, Huynh PD, Thall EH: Altered uptake of infrared diode laser by retina after intravitreal indocyanine green dye and internal limiting membrane peeling. Am J Ophthalmol 2002;134:285–286.
110 Kumar A, Prakash G, Singh RP: Indocyanine green enhanced maculorhexis in macular hole surgery. Indian J Ophthalmol 2002;50:123–126.
111 Kwok AK, Yeung YS, Lee VY, Wong TH: ICG-assisted peeling of the retinal ILM. Ophthalmology 2002;109:1040.
112 Haritoglou C, Gass CA, Gandorfer A, Kampik A: ICG-assisted peeling of the retinal ILM. Ophthalmology 2002;109:1039.
113 Cheung BT, Yuen CY, Lam DS, Tang HM, Yan YN, Chen WQ: ICG-assisted peeling of the retinal ILM. Ophthalmology 2002;109:1039–1040.
114 Engelbrecht NE, Freeman J, Sternberg P, Aaberg TM Jr, Aaberg TM Sr, Martin DF, Sippy BD: Retinal pigment epithelial changes after macular hole surgery with indocyanine green-assisted internal limiting membrane peeling. Am J Ophthalmol 2002;133:89–94.

115 Stalmans P, Parys-Vanginderdeuren R, De Vos R, Feron EJ: ICG staining of the inner limiting membrane facilitates its removal during surgery for macular holes and puckers. Bull Soc Belge Ophtalmol 2001;281:21–26.
116 Da Mata AP, Burk SE, Riemann CD, Rosa RH Jr, Snyder ME, Petersen MR, Foster RE: Indocyanine green-assisted peeling of the retinal internal limiting membrane during vitrectomy surgery for macular hole repair. Ophthalmology 2001;108:1187–1192.
117 Weinberger AW, Kirchhof B, Mazinani BE, Schrage NF: Persistent indocyanine green (ICG) fluorescence 6 weeks after intraocular ICG administration for macular hole surgery. Graefes Arch Clin Exp Ophthalmol 2001;239:388–390.
118 Gandorfer A, Messmer EM, Ulbig MW, Kampik A: Indocyanine green selectively stains the internal limiting membrane. Am J Ophthalmol 2001;131:387–388.
119 Gandorfer A, Haritoglou C, Gass CA, Ulbig MW, Kampik A: Indocyanine green-assisted peeling of the internal limiting membrane may cause retinal damage. Am J Ophthalmol 2001;132:431–433.
120 Haritoglou C, Gandorfer A, Gass CA, Schaumberger M, Ulbig MW, Kampik A: Indocyanine green-assisted peeling of the internal limiting membrane in macular hole surgery affects visual outcome: a clinicopathologic correlation. Am J Ophthalmol 2002; 134:836–841.
121 Ricci F, Pucci S, Sesti F, Missiroli F, Cerulli L, Spagnoli LG: Modulation of Ku70/80, clusterin/ApoJ isoforms and Bax expression in indocyanine-green-mediated photo-oxidative cell damage. Ophthalmic Res 2007;39:164–173.
122 Penha FM, Maia M, Eid Farah M, Principe AH, Freymuller EH, Maia A, Magalhaes O Jr, Smith RL: Effects of subretinal injections of indocyanine green, trypan blue, and glucose in rabbit eyes. Ophthalmology 2007;114:899–908.
123 Ueno A, Hisatomi T, Enaida H, Kagimoto T, Mochizuki Y, Goto Y, Kubota T, Hata Y, Ishibashi T: Biocompatibility of brilliant blue G in a rat model of subretinal injection. Retina 2007;27:499–504.
124 Hirasawa H, Yanagi Y, Tamaki Y, Inoue Y, Kadonosono K: Indocyanine green and trypan blue: intracellular uptake and extracellular binding by human retinal pigment epithelial cells. Retina 2007;27: 375–378.
125 Kunikata H, Tomita H, Abe T, Murata H, Sagara Y, Sato H, Wada Y, Fuse N, Nakagawa Y, Tamai M, Nishida K: Hypothermia protects cultured human retinal pigment epithelial cells against indocyanine green toxicity. J Ocul Pharmacol Ther 2007;23:35–39.
126 Proulx AA, Gonder JR: Comparison of in vitro toxicity of single vs double exposures of indocyanine green in human retinal pigment epithelial cell cultures. Am J Ophthalmol 2007;143:353–354.
127 Saikia P, Maisch T, Kobuch K, Jackson TL, Baumler W, Szeimies RM, Gabel VP, Hillenkamp J: Safety testing of indocyanine green in an ex vivo porcine retina model. Invest Ophthalmol Vis Sci 2006;47: 4998–5003.
128 Skrivanova K, Skorpikova J, Svihalek J, Mornstein V, Janisch R: Photochemical properties of a potential photosensitiser indocyanine green in vitro. J Photochem Photobiol B 2006;85:150–154.
129 Haritoglou C, Freyer W, Priglinger SG, Kampik A: Light absorbing properties of indocyanine green (ICG) in solution and after adsorption to the retinal surface: an ex-vivo approach. Graefes Arch Clin Exp Ophthalmol 2006;244:1196–1202.
130 Schuettauf F, Haritoglou C, May CA, Rejdak R, Mankowska A, Freyer W, Eibl K, Zrenner E, Kampik A, Thaler S: Administration of novel dyes for intraocular surgery: an in vivo toxicity animal study. Invest Ophthalmol Vis Sci 2006;47:3573–3578.
131 Mennel S, Thumann G, Peter S, Meyer CH, Kroll P: Influence of vital dyes on the function of the outer blood-retinal barrier in vitro. Klin Monatsbl Augenheilkd 2006;223:568–576.
132 Goldstein M, Zemel E, Loewenstein A, Perlman I: Retinal toxicity of indocyanine green in albino rabbits. Invest Ophthalmol Vis Sci 2006;47:2100–2107.
133 Sato Y, Tomita H, Sugano E, Isago H, Yoshida M, Tamai M: Evaluation of indocyanine green toxicity to rat retinas. Ophthalmologica 2006;220:153–158.
134 Kiilgaard JF, Nissen MH, la Cour M: An isotonic preparation of 1 mg/ml indocyanine green is not toxic to hyperconfluent ARPE19 cells, even after prolonged exposure. Acta Ophthalmol Scand 2006; 84:42–46.
135 Yip HK, Lai TY, So KF, Kwok AK: Retinal ganglion cells toxicity caused by photosensitising effects of intravitreal indocyanine green with illumination in rat eyes. Br J Ophthalmol 2006;90:99–102.
136 Ikagawa H, Yoneda M, Iwaki M, Isogai Z, Tsujii K, Yamazaki R, Kamiya T, Zako M: Chemical toxicity of indocyanine green damages retinal pigment epithelium. Invest Ophthalmol Vis Sci 2005;46:2531–2539.
137 Gandorfer A, Rohleder M, Charteris DG, Sethi C, Kampik A, Luthert P: Staining and peeling of the internal limiting membrane in the cat eye. Curr Eye Res 2005;30:977–987.
138 Jin Y, Uchida S, Yanagi Y, Aihara M, Araie M: Neurotoxic effects of trypan blue on rat retinal ganglion cells. Exp Eye Res 2005;81:395–400.
139 Kodjikian L, Richter T, Halberstadt M, Beby F, Flueckiger F, Boehnke M, Garweg JG: Toxic effects of indocyanine green, infracyanine green, and trypan blue on the human retinal pigmented epithelium. Graefes Arch Clin Exp Ophthalmol 2005;243: 917–925.

140 Melendez RF, Kumar N, Maswadi SM, Zaslow K, Glickmank RD: Photodynamic actions of indocyanine green and trypan blue on human lens epithelial cells in vitro. Am J Ophthalmol 2005;140:132–134.
141 Kwok AK, Lai TY, Yeung CK, Yeung YS, Li WW, Chiang SW: The effects of indocyanine green and endoillumination on rabbit retina: an electroretinographic and histological study. Br J Ophthalmol 2005;89:897–900.
142 Narayanan R, Kenney MC, Kamjoo S, Trinh TH, Seigel GM, Resende GP, Kuppermann BD: Toxicity of indocyanine green (ICG) in combination with light on retinal pigment epithelial cells and neurosensory retinal cells. Curr Eye Res 2005;30:471–478.
143 Chang YS, Tseng SY, Tseng SH, Chen YT, Hsiao JH: Comparison of dyes for cataract surgery. 1. Cytotoxicity to corneal endothelial cells in a rabbit model. J Cataract Refract Surg 2005;31:792–798.
144 Chang AA, Zhu M, Billson F: The interaction of indocyanine green with human retinal pigment epithelium. Invest Ophthalmol Vis Sci 2005;46: 1463–1467.
145 Haritoglou C, Priglinger S, Gandorfer A, Welge-Lussen U, Kampik A: Histology of the vitreoretinal interface after indocyanine green staining of the ILM, with illumination using a halogen and xenon light source. Invest Ophthalmol Vis Sci 2005;46: 1468–1472.
146 Murata M, Shimizu S, Horiuchi S, Sato S: The effect of indocyanine green on cultured retinal glial cells. Retina 2005;25:75–80.
147 Chao AN, Chen SN, Kuo YH: Retinal function and histologic changes following intravitreal injection of indocyanine green in a rabbit model. J Ocul Pharmacol Ther 2004;20:450–459.
148 Jackson TL, Vote B, Knight BC, El-Amir A, Stanford MR, Marshall J: Safety testing of infracyanine green using retinal pigment epithelium and glial cell cultures. Invest Ophthalmol Vis Sci 2004;45:3697–3703.
149 Wu WC, Hu DN, Roberts JE: Phototoxicity of indocyanine green on human retinal pigment epithelium in vitro and its reduction by lutein. Photochem Photobiol 2004, E-pub ahead of print.
150 Jackson TL, Hillenkamp J, Knight BC, Zhang JJ, Thomas D, Stanford MR, Marshall J: Safety testing of indocyanine green and trypan blue using retinal pigment epithelium and glial cell cultures. Invest Ophthalmol Vis Sci 2004;45:2778–2785.
151 Hsu SL, Kao YH, Wu WC: Effect of indocyanine green on the growth and viability of cultured human retinal pigment epithelial cells. J Ocul Pharmacol Ther 2004;20:353–362.
152 Wollensak G, Spoerl E, Wirbelauer C, Pham DT: Influence of indocyanine green staining on the biomechanical strength of porcine internal limiting membrane. Ophthalmologica 2004;218:278–282.
153 Gale JS, Proulx AA, Gonder JR, Mao AJ, Hutnik CM: Comparison of the in vitro toxicity of indocyanine green to that of trypan blue in human retinal pigment epithelium cell cultures. Am J Ophthalmol 2004;138:64–69.
154 Ho JD, Chen HC, Chen SN, Tsai RJ: Reduction of indocyanine green-associated photosensitizing toxicity in retinal pigment epithelium by sodium elimination. Arch Ophthalmol 2004;122:871–878.
155 Rezai KA, Farrokh-Siar L, Ernest JT, van Seventer GA: Indocyanine green induces apoptosis in human retinal pigment epithelial cells. Am J Ophthalmol 2004;137:931–933.
156 Tokuda K, Tsukamoto T, Fujisawa S, Matsubara M: Evaluation of toxicity due to vital stains in isolated rat retinas. Acta Ophthalmol Scand 2004;82: 189–194.
157 Ho JD, Tsai RJ, Chen SN, Chen HC: Removal of sodium from the solvent reduces retinal pigment epithelium toxicity caused by indocyanine green: implications for macular hole surgery. Br J Ophthalmol 2004;88:556–559.
158 Czajka MP, McCuen BW 2nd, Cummings TJ, Nguyen H, Stinnett S, Wong F: Effects of indocyanine green on the retina and retinal pigment epithelium in a porcine model of retinal hole. Retina 2004;24: 275–282.
159 Iriyama A, Uchida S, Yanagi Y, Tamaki Y, Inoue Y, Matsuura K, Kadonosono K, Araie M: Effects of indocyanine green on retinal ganglion cells. Invest Ophthalmol Vis Sci 2004;45:943–947.
160 Haritoglou C, Gandorfer A, Gass CA, Kampik A: Histology of the vitreoretinal interface after staining of the internal limiting membrane using glucose 5% diluted indocyanine and infracyanine green. Am J Ophthalmol 2004;137:345–348.
161 Maia M, Margalit E, Lakhanpal R, Tso MO, Grebe R, Torres G, Au Eong KG, Farah ME, Fujii GY, Weiland J, de Juan E Jr, D'Anna SA, Humayun MS: Effects of intravitreal indocyanine green injection in rabbits. Retina 2004;24:69–79.
162 Kawaji T, Hirata A, Inomata Y, Koga T, Tanihara H: Morphological damage in rabbit retina caused by subretinal injection of indocyanine green. Graefes Arch Clin Exp Ophthalmol 2004;242:158–164.
163 Grisanti S, Szurman P, Gelisken F, Aisenbrey S, Oficjalska-Mlynczak J, Bartz-Schmidt KU: Histological findings in experimental macular surgery with indocyanine green. Invest Ophthalmol Vis Sci 2004; 45:282–286.
164 Lee JE, Yoon TJ, Oum BS, Lee JS, Choi HY: Toxicity of indocyanine green injected into the subretinal space: subretinal toxicity of indocyanine green. Retina 2003;23:675–681.

165 Ho JD, Tsai RJ, Chen SN, Chen HC: Cytotoxicity of indocyanine green on retinal pigment epithelium: implications for macular hole surgery. Arch Ophthalmol 2003;121:1423–1429.
166 Paques M, Genevois O, Regnier A, Tadayoni R, Sercombe R, Gaudric A, Vicaut E: Axon-tracing properties of indocyanine green. Arch Ophthalmol 2003;121:367–370.
167 Dietz FB, Jaffe RA: Indocyanine green: evidence of neurotoxicity in spinal root axons. Anesthesiology 2003;98:516–520.
168 Yam HF, Kwok AK, Chan KP, Lai TY, Chu KY, Lam DS, Pang CP: Effect of indocyanine green and illumination on gene expression in human retinal pigment epithelial cells. Invest Ophthalmol Vis Sci 2003;44:370–377.
169 Gandorfer A, Haritoglou C, Gandorfer A, Kampik A: Retinal damage from indocyanine green in experimental macular surgery. Invest Ophthalmol Vis Sci 2003;44:316–323.
170 Nakamura T, Murata T, Hisatomi T, Enaida H, Sassa Y, Ueno A, Sakamoto T, Ishibashi T: Ultrastructure of the vitreoretinal interface following the removal of the internal limiting membrane using indocyanine green. Curr Eye Res 2003;27:395–399.
171 Enaida H, Sakamoto T, Hisatomi T, Goto Y, Ishibashi T: Morphological and functional damage of the retina caused by intravitreous indocyanine green in rat eyes. Graefes Arch Clin Exp Ophthalmol 2002; 240:209–213.
172 Holley GP, Alam A, Kiri A, Edelhauser HF: Effect of indocyanine green intraocular stain on human and rabbit corneal endothelial structure and viability. An in vitro study. J Cataract Refract Surg 2002;28: 1027–1033.
173 Burk SE, Da Mata AP, Snyder ME, Rosa RH Jr, Foster RE: Indocyanine green-assisted peeling of the retinal internal limiting membrane. Ophthalmology 2000; 107:2010–2014.
174 Varriale L, Crescenzi E, Paba V, di Celso BM, Palumbo G: Selective light-induced modulation of bcl-XL and bax expressions in indocyanine green-loaded U937 cells: effects of continuous or intermittent photo-sensitization with low IR-light using a 805-nm diode laser. J Photochem Photobiol B 2000; 57:66–75.
175 Abels C, Fickweiler S, Weiderer P, Baumler W, Hofstadter F, Landthaler M, Szeimies RM: Indocyanine green (ICG) and laser irradiation induce photooxidation. Arch Dermatol Res 2000;292:404–411.
176 Baumler W, Abels C, Karrer S, Weiss T, Messmann H, Landthaler M, Szeimies RM: Photo-oxidative killing of human colonic cancer cells using indocyanine green and infrared light. Br J Cancer 1999;80: 360–363.
177 Chang AA, Morse LS, Handa JT, Morales RB, Tucker R, Hjelmeland L, Yannuzzi LA: Histologic localization of indocyanine green dye in aging primate and human ocular tissues with clinical angiographic correlation. Ophthalmology 1998;105:1060–1068.
178 Fickweiler S, Szeimies RM, Baumler W, Steinbach P, Karrer S, Goetz AE, Abels C, Hofstadter F, Landthaler M: Indocyanine green: intracellular uptake and phototherapeutic effects in vitro. J Photochem Photobiol B 1997;38:178–183.
179 Sakamoto H, Yamanaka I, Kubota T, Ishibashi T: Indocyanine green-assisted peeling of the epiretinal membrane in proliferative vitreoretinopathy. Graefes Arch Clin Exp Ophthalmol 2003;241:204–207.
180 Kwok AK, Li WW, Pang CP, Lai TY, Yam GH, Chan NR, Lam DS: Indocyanine green staining and removal of internal limiting membrane in macular hole surgery: histology and outcome. Am J Ophthalmol 2001;132:178–183.
181 Kroemer I, Lommatzsch A, Pauleikhoff D: Retinal ICG-accumulation after ILM-staining during macular hole surgery? Ophthalmologe 2004;101:604–607.
182 Brazitikos PD, Androudi S, Tsinopoulos I, Papadopoulos NT, Balidis M, Georgiadis N: Functional and anatomic results of macular hole surgery complicated by massive indocyanine green subretinal migration. Acta Ophthalmol Scand 2004; 82: 613–615.
183 Yam GHF, Kwok AK, Chan KP, Lai TY, Lam DS, Pang CP: Effect off indocyanine green and illumination on gene expression in human retinal pigment epithelial cells. Invest Ophthalmol Vis Sci 2004;44:370–377.
184 Landsman ML, Kwant G, Mook GA, Zijlstra WG: Light-absorbing properties, stability and spectral stabilization of indocyanine green. J Appl Physiol 1976;40:575–583.
185 Zhou JF, Chin MP, Schafer SA: Aggregation and degradation of indocyanine green; in Anderson R (ed): Laser Surgery: Advanced Characterization, Therapeutics and Systems IV. Bellingham, SPIE, 1994, pp 495–499.
186 Benz MS, Smiddy WE: Increased diode laser uptake in inner retinal layers after indocyanine green staining of the internal limiting membrane. Ophthalmic Surg Lasers Imaging 2003;34:64–67.
187 Fickweiler S, Szeimies RM, Baumler W, Steinbach P, Karrer S, Goetz AE, Abels C, Hofstadter F, Landthaler M: Indocyanine green: intracellular uptake and phototherapeutic effects in vitro. J Photochem Photobiol B 1997;38:178–183.
188 Fuller D, Machemer R, Knighton RW: Retinal damage produced by intraocular fiber optic light. Am J Ophthalmol 1978;85:519–537.

189 Meyers SM, Bonner RF: Retinal irradiance from vitrectomy endoilluminators. Am J Ophthalmol 1982; 94:26–29.

190 Kadonosono K, Takeuchi S, Yabuki K, Yamakawa T, Mekada A, Uchio E: Absorption of short wavelengths of endoillumination in indocyanine green solution: implications for internal limiting membrane removal. Graefes Arch Clin Exp Ophthalmol 2003;241:284–286.

191 Sippy BD, Engelbrecht NE, Hubbard GB, Moriarty SE, Jiang S, Aaberg TM Jr, Aaberg TM Sr, Grossniklaus HE, Sternberg P: Indocyanine green effect on cultured human retinal pigment epithelial cells: implication for macular hole surgery. Am J Ophthalmol 2001;132:433–435.

192 Stalmans P, van Aken EH, Veckeneer M, Feron EJ, Stalmans I: Toxic effect of indocyanine green on retinal pigment epithelium related to osmotic effects of the solvent. Am J Ophthalmol 2002:134:282–285.

Prof. Salvatore Grisanti, MD
Department of Ophthalmology, University of Luebeck
Ratzeburger Allee 160
DE–23538 Luebeck (Germany)
Tel. +49 451 500 2210, Fax +49 451 500 3085, E-Mail salvatore.grisanti@uk-sh.de

Meyer CH (ed): Vital Dyes in Vitreoretinal Surgery.
Dev Ophthalmol. Basel, Karger, 2008, vol 42, pp 69–81

Toxicity of Indocyanine Green in Vitreoretinal Surgery

Arnd Gandorfer · Christos Haritoglou · Anselm Kampik

Department of Ophthalmology, Ludwig-Maximilians-University, Munich, Germany

Abstract

Indocyanine green (ICG) selectively stains the internal limiting membrane (ILM) of the retina, and helps to visualize and remove the membrane from the retina. Toxicity and damage to the retina has been reported in in vitro and in vivo studies, and following macular surgery. Toxic effects can occur to retinal glial cells, to the nerve fiber layer, to retinal ganglion cells, and to the optic nerve. In case of subretinal application, the retinal pigment epithelium can be affected. The mechanisms of toxicity are unclear. Whether the dye itself or some preparations only are causing harm to the retina is subject of an ongoing debate. ICG changes the light absorption properties of the ILM and enhances the stiffness of the membrane, probably by cross-linking of collagen fibers. Beside better visualization, this effect is responsible for the ease of membrane removal compared to unaided ILM peeling. Whether a phototoxic effect, which has been demonstrated in vitro and in vivo, plays a clinically significant role in macular surgery has neither been proven nor ruled out yet. ICG at concentrations higher than 1.25% or application of the dye in air are very likely causing retinal damage. In addition, lower concentrations also carry the risk of iatrogenic damage, depending on the final concentration of potentially toxic substances at the vitreomacular interface and on other mechanisms. Due to its instability and the unpredictable effects of ICG at the macula, it cannot be recommended for clinical use before its safety has been proven. This chapter reviews the literature related to ICG toxicity, and summarizes dye-related untoward effects in postmortem eyes and ex vivo models, in in vitro and in vivo animal models, and in macular surgery.

Indocyanine green (ICG) is a water-soluble dye with a peak absorption at around 800 nm and a peak emission at 835 nm. Its molecular weight is 775 Da, and the formula ($C_{43}H_{47}N_2NaO_6S_2$) is shown in figure 1. Before its ophthalmic application, ICG was used for assessment of cardiac output, liver blood flow, and hepatic function. ICG contains iodine, and is unstable in aqueous solution.

ICG powder should be dissolved with the aqueous solvent provided by the manufacturer: 10 ml of aqueous solvent is added to 25 mg ICG to achieve a concentration of 2.5 mg/ml. After shaking, it can be further diluted with balanced salt solution (BSS); for example, 0.5 ml of this solution is diluted with 0.5 ml BSS for a concentration of 1.25 mg/ml.

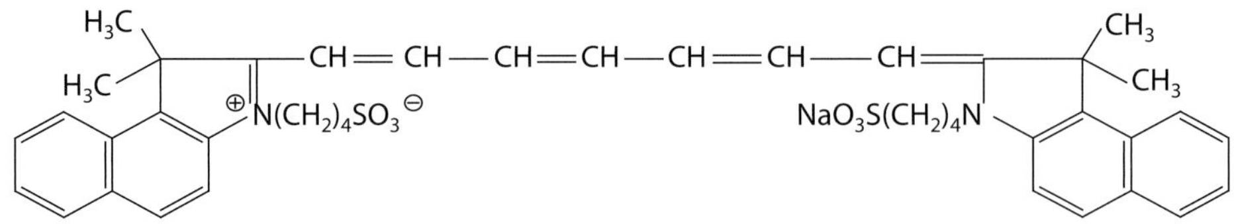

Fig. 1. Formula of ICG.

ICG dye selectively stains the internal limiting membrane (ILM) of the retina [1–3]. The contrast between the green-stained ILM and the unstained underlying retina facilitates initiation of the peel and enables precise monitoring of its extent. In addition, ICG dye allows safe identification of residual vitreous cortex by the lack of staining, and enables the surgeon to remove cortical vitreous remnants more completely in areas of vitreoschisis [1, 4].

As many other vitreoretinal surgeons we started using ICG in the year 2000. Our initial enthusiasm waned, however, when routine transmission electron microscopy of ILM specimens revealed removed retinal structures, and functional results were unfavorable compared to unaided peeling [5–9]. These observations were in contrast to our experience in terms of surgical outcome and pathology workup documented previously [10, 11]. We abandoned ICG, and ultrastructural findings and functional results returned to normal [12]. Of note, no other change in the surgical setting took place, and it was clear that ICG was responsible for these observations [13].

Since that time, a possible toxic effect of ICG on the retina has become the subject of an ongoing debate. There is a growing number of articles dealing with ICG-related toxicity in vitro and in vivo. In macular surgery, several authors have shown significant visual field defects and less favorable results in visual acuity when ICG was used intraoperatively, whereas others have reported good functional outcome of ICG-assisted vitrectomy.

This chapter is focused on the current knowledge of ICG-related toxicity, and will report on postmortem findings, as well as in vitro, in vivo, and ex vivo models simulating the application of ICG in macular surgery. In addition, a brief summary of the literature of ICG-assisted ILM peeling in macular surgery is given.

Postmortem Findings

Given the contrast between removal of retinal structures after ICG-assisted peeling and conventional peeling, we performed several experiments in human postmortem eyes [14]. The vitreous was removed, and the ILM was stained with 0.05% ICG. In some eyes, the retina was additionally illuminated, and the emission spectra were modified by using blocking filters. In brief, exposure of ICG-stained ILM to wavelengths beyond 620 nm resulted in severe damage to the inner retina, including loss of the ILM, cellular disorganization, and fragmentation of the cytoplasm. ICG staining alone or in combination with wavelengths of 380–620 nm disclosed rupture of Müller cells with detachment of the ILM, but no other cellular disorganization. Eyes subjected to illumination only showed no abnormalities. We concluded that ICG alone led to ILM detachment caused by Müller cell rupture at their basal membrane side, and in addition, there was a wavelength-related effect of the photosensitive dye ICG [14].

In a companion article, we reported on the light-absorbing properties and the osmolarity of ICG depending on the concentration and the solvent medium [15]. We found that dilution of ICG using BSS or BSS plus resulted in a steep increase in absorption starting at 600 nm. The absorption band of ICG diluted in viscoelastic material was similar to the saline solution-diluted ICG. As peak absorption at 700 nm forming a shoulder in the absorption curve, decreased at lower concentrations (0.001 or 0.00025% ICG), and the absorption peak around 780–800 nm remained stable, we concluded that the overlap between the absorption band of ICG and the emission spectrum of the light source was especially critical with higher concentrations of ICG such as 0.05 or 0.5%, which were commonly used in macular surgery at that time. Osmolarity, which was accused of causing retinal damage at the beginning of ICG-assisted vitrectomy, was in the range of 302–313 mosm for BSS-plus-diluted ICG and 292–298 mosm when glucose 5% was used for dilution [15].

We went on assessing the effect of ICG and infracyanine green diluted with glucose 5%. Both solutions caused significant morphologic alterations of the inner retina after light exposure, and no difference was noted between the two products [16].

Then, we modified the light source and investigated species-related differences [17]. We applied a high concentration of ICG (0.5%) to the ILM of human donor eyes and to porcine eyes followed by illumination using a halogen and a xenon light source. Only the combination of the halogen light source and ICG caused retinal damage in human eyes. In the xenon light group, there was only slight vacuolization of the inner retina. In porcine eyes, no impact attributable to the light source or ICG alone was noted [17]. This confirmed previous findings by Grisanti et al. [18] which were in contrast to our results in human eyes. Obviously, the porcine eye is less susceptible to ICG damage compared with the human eye.

In vitro Studies

Kodjikian et al. [19] incubated monolayers of human retinal pigment epithelium (RPE) cells with three different concentrations of ICG (0.005, 0.05, 0.5%). They observed acute toxicity after 5 min, and chronic toxicity after 6 days at a concentration above

0.05%. This was also seen when iodine-free infracyanine green was used instead of ICG [19].

Ikagawa et al. [20] have shown that ICG functions as a unique precipitating factor which renders the soluble molecules in serum that are indispensable in the culture of RPE cells insoluble during a 12-hour exposure, resulting in poor cell survival in vitro.

Murata et al. [21] exposed rat retinal glial cells in culture to ICG concentrations of 0.05 and 0.5%. ICG significantly decreased the viable cell number of retinal glial cells at the high concentration, whereas no such effect was seen at the lower concentration. As bcl-2 mRNA levels were higher in cells treated with 0.5% ICG solution, the authors concluded that apoptosis-related signal pathways might play a role [21].

Jin et al. [22] investigated the effect of ICG on rat retinal ganglion cells in culture, and found a time-dependent damage of cells treated with ICG (1.5 mg/ml) solution for 10 s to 30 min.

Narayanan et al. [23] treated human RPE cells (ARPE-19) and rat neurosensory retinal cells (R28) with four different concentrations of ICG (0.015, 0.03, 0.06, and 0.125%) and light. In both cell lines, mitochondrial dehydrogenase activity was decreased and DNA synthesis in retinal cells was increased, pointing towards cell toxicity and dysfunction. The duration of light was an additional significant factor in ICG toxicity [23].

Yam et al. [24] have demonstrated that the application of ICG together with light resulted in a concentration-dependent reduction in RPE cell viability and increased expressions of apoptosis-related genes p53 and *bax* as well as the cell cycle arrest protein p21 in human cultured RPE cells. No such reduction was found in RPE cells treated with ICG without illumination [24].

Jackson et al. [25] have shown that application of ICG with illumination resulted in a significant reduction in cell viability in glial cell culture compared with cells treated with ICG without illumination.

In vivo Studies

Intravitreal Injection of Indocyanine Green in Rat Eyes

In 2001, Enaida et al. [26] injected ICG into the rat vitreous after gas-induced vitrectomy 2 weeks earlier. They found retinal damage in light microscopy at doses of 25 and 2.5 mg/ml ICG. Even at low doses, such as 0.25 or 0.025 mg/ml, there was functional impairment in the electroretinogram (ERG) [26].

Schuettauf et al. [27] injected several dyes into the vitreous cavity of rat eyes, including ICG 0.0002–0.5%. Eight eyes were treated with each concentration. Seven days thereafter, all eyes with 0.5% ICG showed degenerative changes in histological workup, and the inner retina was significantly thinner compared to BSS-injected control eyes. No such alterations were seen with 0.002% and with 0.0002%

ICG. However, retinal ganglion cell count was significantly reduced at all tested concentrations [27].

Iriyama et al. [28] also found a significant decrease in the number of viable rat retinal ganglion cells 14 days after intravitreal injection of ICG at a concentration of 2.5 mg/ml. In a companion experiment, they briefly exposed rat retinal ganglion cells to this concentration of ICG in vitro, followed by incubation for 3 days. A dose-dependent reduction in viable retinal ganglion cells was found, pointing towards a direct toxicity of ICG to retinal ganglion cells [28].

Sato et al. [29] reported on degeneration of all retinal layers in the central retinal area following an intravitreal injection of a relatively high dose concentration of ICG (5 or 25 mg/ml) in rat eyes. In these areas of damage, glutamine synthetase immunoreactivity was decreased as a sign of Müller cell dysfunction. In addition, they found a decrease in viability of cultured RPE cells depending on the ICG dose [29].

Yip et al. [30] injected rat eyes with 1.0 ml/mg ICG solution and additionally applied illumination. Eyes injected with ICG without illumination showed an insignificant reduction in retinal ganglion cell density compared with the control group, whereas a significant decrease in retinal ganglion cell density was found in eyes that had ICG injection and illumination. The density of retinal ganglion cells was determined with retrograde labelling 1 month after intravitreal injection [30].

Intravitreal Injection of Indocyanine Green in Rabbit Eyes

Maia et al. [31] investigated the effect of three different concentrations of ICG (0.5, 5, and 25 mg/ml) in rabbit eyes. 0.1 ml ICG was injected into the rabbit vitreous. In brief, alteration in ERG responses and morphological retinal damage was observed, proportional to increasing ICG concentrations [31].

Chao et al. [32] injected 0.1 ml of different ICG concentrations (0.5, 0.1 mg/ml) into the rabbit vitreous. They also found ERG and morphological alterations in a dose- and time-dependent manner [32].

In a third study, Goldstein et al. [33] found damage to all retinal layers and permanent functional impairment in albino rabbit eyes treated with 0.1 ml ICG (2.5 mg/ml) intravitreally.

Vitrectomy, Indocyanine Green Application, and Endoillumination

Kwok et al. [34] performed vitrectomy followed by ICG application (0.1 ml ICG at 2.5 mg/ml) for 30 s and 10 min of endoillumination. Significant ERG changes and outer retinal damage was seen after 1 week of follow-up [34].

Subretinal Injection of Indocyanine Green in Rabbit Eyes

Maia et al. [35] reported on RPE, photoreceptor inner and outer segment, and outer nuclear layer damage in rabbit eyes after subretinal injection of ICG at a concentration of 5 mg/ml. Lee et al. [36] also found outer retinal damage after subretinal injection of ICG at concentrations of 1.25 mg/ml or higher. Finally, Kawaji et al. [37] confirmed the dependence of outer retinal damage on ICG concentration after subretinal ICG application.

Vitrectomy and Internal Limiting Membrane Staining in Cat Eyes

We performed vitrectomy and ILM staining in a cat model [38]. 0.5% ICG was applied to the retinal surface for 1 min, and then washed out. Additional endoillumination for 3 min followed. The results from ICG staining alone and from ICG staining with illumination were compared. It is of note that no attempt at peeling was made. ICG staining of the cat ILM resulted in detachment of the ILM from the retina (fig. 2). In transmission electron microscopy, there was a continuous layer of adherent retinal structures, such as Müller cell fragments. The Müller cells were ruptured at their basal membrane side. Additional illumination caused severe inner retinal damage, such as loss of the ILM and disintegration of retinal cytoarchitecture (fig. 3). The results of this in vivo study confirmed our findings obtained in postmortem eyes with respect to toxicity of ICG alone and in combination with illumination [38].

Nakamura et al. [39] performed ICG-assisted ILM peeling in primates. They describe and illustrate tearing of Müller cells and total removal of Müller cell end feet with consequent exposure of the nerve fiber layer to the vitreous fluid in the peeled area [39]. The retinal debris adherent to the retinal side of the ILM presented in their study is very similar to our findings in human ILM specimens after ICG-assisted ILM removal in vivo and in specimens from experimental ICG-assisted surgery in human donor eyes, and it appears to us that the damage observed is more attributable to ICG than to peeling itself [40].

Ex vivo Models

Tokuda et al. [41] reported on marked morphological damage to isolated rat retina exposed to ICG 0.5% solution, and significantly higher lactate dehydrogenase activities measured in the medium.

Saikia et al. [42] assessed ICG in a porcine ex vivo perfusion organ culture model. ICG 1% dissolved in glucose 5% induced apoptosis but not necrosis. No apoptosis was seen with brief exposure to ICG 0.1% for 1 min and illumination for 3 min. Of note, ICG applied briefly to the retinal surface gradually penetrated the entire retina [42].

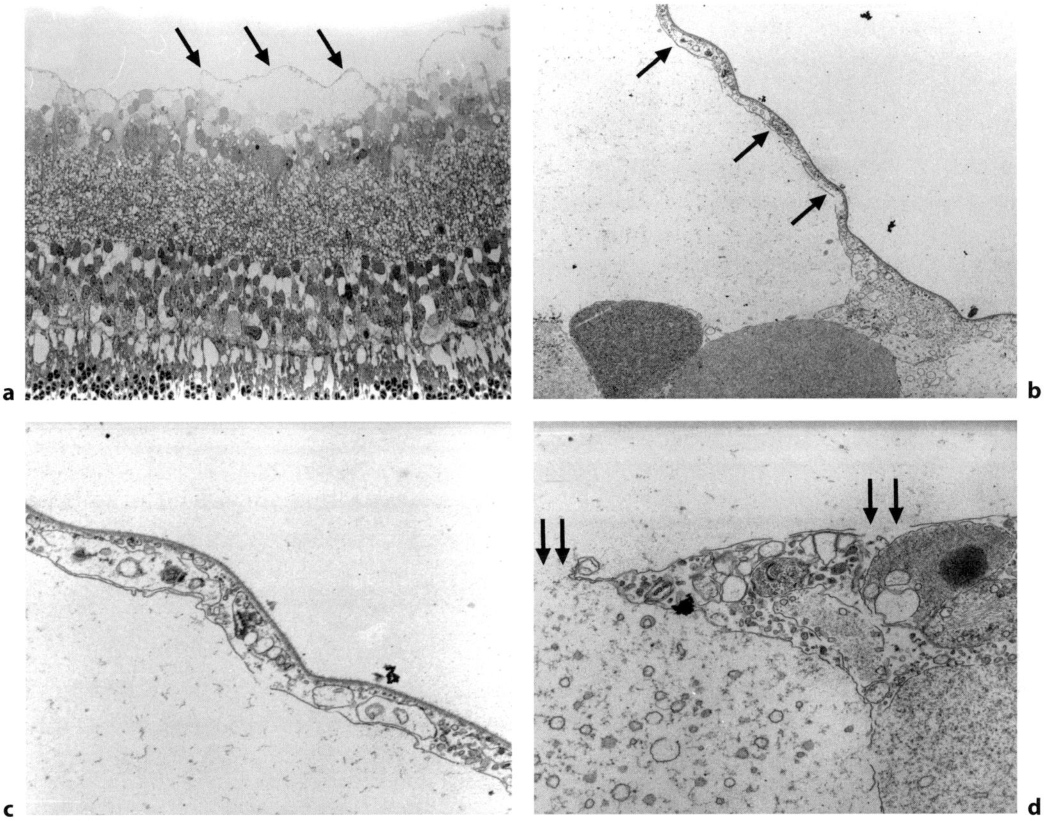

Fig. 2. ICG staining of the cat ILM. **a** Light micrograph showing focal detachments of the ILM (arrows). **b** Transmission electron micrograph demonstrating detachment of the ILM with a continuous layer of adherent retinal structures (arrows). **c** Higher magnification of **b**. Müller cell fragments cover the retinal side of the ILM as a continuous band. **d** Tearing of Müller cell end feet. Arrows indicate ruptured cell membrane. Magnifications: ×400 (**a**); ×4,800 (**b**); ×9,600 (**c**, **d**). Reprint with permission from Gandorfer et al. [38].

Wollensak et al. [43] stained the ILM of porcine retina with 0.005% ICG followed by illumination at 400–800 nm for 3 min. Biomechanical force elongation measurements were performed using an automated material tester. They found a significant increase in ultimate force by 45% and a decrease in elongation by 24%. It was concluded that a photosensitizing effect of ICG led to collagen cross-linking resulting in an increase in the biomechanical stiffness of the ILM [43]. Similar results were reported when the lens capsule of pig eyes was stained with ICG [44].

Our group investigated the light-absorbing properties of ICG in solution and after adsorption to the retinal surface [45]. On the retinal surface, absorption spectra exhibited a steep increase in absorption beginning at 620 nm, with a maximum at 736 nm (0.05% ICG), a shoulder at 745 nm (0.15% ICG) and a second maximum at

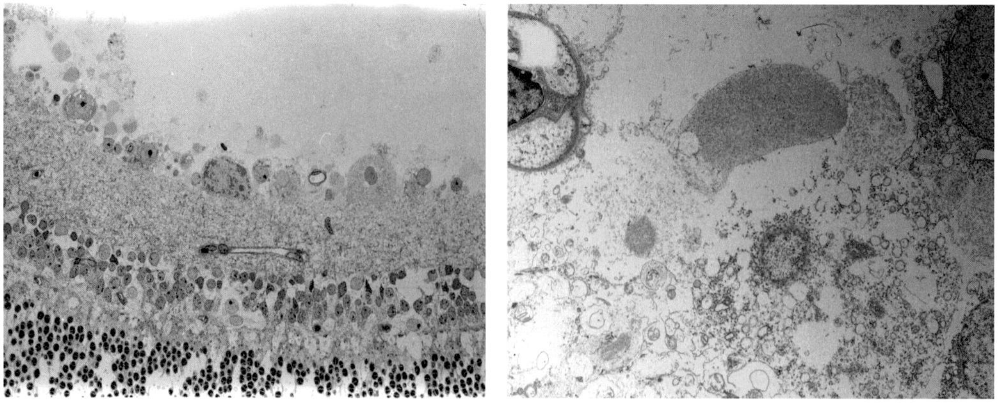

Fig. 3. ICG staining followed by halogen light illumination. **a** Severe inner retinal damage, such as loss of the ILM and disintegration of retinal cytoarchitecture. **b** Transmission electron micrograph demonstrating loss of cellular integrity and undetermined retinal debris. Magnifications: ×400 (**a**); ×9,600 (**b**). Reprint with permission from Gandorfer et al. [38].

around 800 nm for both concentrations. Repeated measurement of the retinal surface 13 days after the ICG exposure revealed no changes in the position of the maxima as compared to the initial measurements. In contrast, ICG dissolved in water or BSS plus disclosed variations in absorption characteristics depending on dye concentration, solute, and time of measurement [45].

In a yet unpublished experiment, we stained the vitreoretinal interface of human donor eyes with 0.05% ICG and 0.06% trypan blue. Laser burns were applied to the unstained and stained macula using a green (532 nm) and an infrared (810 nm) diode laser. The temperature rise in each setting was recorded using a noncontact thermal video system. Light and electron microscopy of retinal specimens was performed, and light absorption of trypan blue and ICG was measured by spectrophotometry. Laser treatment of unstained retina resulted in a temperature rise of 6.3 ± 0.86°C (mean ± standard deviation) with 532 nm, and 4.6 ± 0.48°C with 810 nm, respectively. Application of 810 nm to the trypan-blue-stained retina caused a temperature rise of 9.3 ± 1.6°C. Green laser application (532 nm) resulted in a temperature rise of 15.0 ± 2.8°C, and of 13.6 ± 2.0°C in the trypan-blue-stained and the ICG-stained eye, respectively. In contrast, infrared diode laser application to the ICG-stained ILM caused a temperature rise of 61.3 ± 7.6°C. Microscopy of this specimen showed tissue loss within the inner retina, whereas the other specimens had normal morphology. We concluded from the experiment that the combination of ICG and infrared diode laser results in a marked temperature rise which may cause inner retinal damage due to altered uptake of laser energy by the ICG-stained retina.

Indocyanine-Green-Assisted Internal Limiting Membrane Peeling

There are various reports in the literature on ICG application during macular surgery. Many authors state that ICG is useful and safe for ILM staining [46–56]. Most series are retrospective or observational case series. There are no safety data obtained from a controlled randomized clinical trial comparing ICG-assisted ILM peeling versus unaided peeling. There is no doubt that ICG is useful. The conclusion that it is safe, however, cannot be drawn from any study at present.

There are a number of articles reporting on adverse effects of ICG (table 1). The damage observed is related to the inner retina [5, 7, 8, 57, 58], to the nerve fiber layer and the ganglion cells [59–63], and to the RPE [61, 64–67]. In a recent article, Sekiryu and Iida [68] have shown by using infrared fluorescence that ICG can persist in the eye over years, confirming previous observations [68, 69]. Tadayoni et al. [70] postulated that residual dye staining the inner retina and the nerve fiber layer may cause an anterograde diffusion of ICG into the optic nerve, and this hypothesis was confirmed in animal experiments by Paques et al. [71].

The inconsistent effects of ICG on visual outcome reported in the literature may reflect the differences in concentrations of dye and duration of exposure, and probably, in addition, different damaging pathways of ICG, caused by its instability, poor solubility, degradation products, and light absorption characteristics.

Summary and Conclusion

ICG selectively stains the ILM of the retina, and helps to visualize and remove the membrane. Damage to the retina has been reported in in vitro and in vivo studies. It can occur to retinal glial cells, to the nerve fiber layer, retinal ganglion cells and the optic nerve, as well as combined to all structures of the inner retina. In case of subretinal application, the RPE can be affected. Residual ICG remains in the eye for years.

The mechanisms of toxicity are still unclear. It cannot be determined at present whether the dye itself or some preparations only are causing harm to the retina. ICG changes the light absorption properties of the ILM and enhances the stiffness of the membrane, probably by cross-linking of collagen fibers. Beside better visualization, this effect is responsible for the ease of membrane removal compared to unaided ILM peeling. Whether a phototoxic effect, which has been demonstrated in vitro and in vivo, plays a clinically significant role in macular surgery has neither been proven nor ruled out yet.

ICG concentrations higher than 1.25% or application of the dye in air are very likely causing damage and must not be used in macular surgery. However, lower concentrations also carry the risk of iatrogenic damage, depending on the final concentration of potentially toxic substances at the vitreomacular interface and on other mechanisms which are still poorly understood. Due to its instability and the unpredictable effects of ICG at the macula, it cannot be recommended for clinical use before its safety has been proven.

Table 1. ICG-related toxicity in macular surgery

Reference	Disease	Indocyanine green					Adverse event
		concentration %	volume ml	solvent water +	application	time s	
Kwok et al. [57]	IMH (10)	0.025	ND	BSS		30	retinal elements adherent to the ILM in histology
Stalmans et al. [58]	IMH (4)	0.33	0.1–0.3	glucose 5%		180	glial cell-like processes adherent to ILM
Gandorfer et al. [5]	IMH (10)	0.5	0.2	BSS		immediate removal	Müller cell footplates adherent to ILM
Engelbrecht et al. [64]	IMH (21)	0.1	1–2	BSS		30–150	RPE changes in 55%
Haritoglou et al. [7]	IMH (20)	0.05	0.2–0.5	BSS		60	retinal debris adherent to ILM, nasal visual field defects
Haritoglou et al. [9]	ERM (20)	0.05	up to 0.5	BSS		60	loss of lines in 35%, visual field defects in 35%, retinal structures adherent to ILM
Wolf et al. [65]	IMH (37)	0.25	0.25	BSS		immediate removal	RPE changes in 27%
Uemura et al. [59]	ERM (16)	0.5	0.6–0.8	BSS		180	visual field defects in 57%
Ando et al. [60]	DME (15)	0.5	0.1–0.2	BSS		immediate removal	optic nerve atrophy in 47%
Cheng et al. [61]	IMH (5) PVR (1)	0.25	1.5	BSS		120	RPE atrophy, optic nerve atrophy
Posselt et al. [66]	IMH (14)	0.5	0.2–0.4	BSS		60–180	RPE changes in 50%
Tognetto et al. [67]	ERM (1)	0.05	ND	glucose 5%	ICG on bare retina after ERM removal	immediate removal	macular edema and RPE changes
Ueno et al. [62]	IMH (16) ERM (14)	0.25	ND	BSS	ICG in air	immediate removal	ERG reduction in photopic negative response
Lai et al. [63]	ERM (13)	0.5 and 1.25	0.2	BSS	ICG in air after ERM peeling	30	N1 and P1 response reduction in multifocal ERG after 1.25% ICG

IMH = Idiopathic macular hole; ND = not determined; ERM = epiretinal membrane; DME = diabetic macular edema; PVR = proliferative vitreoretinopathy. Figures in parentheses indicate number of eyes.

References

1 Gandorfer A, Messmer EM, Ulbig MW, Kampik A: Indocyanine green selectively stains the internal limiting membrane. Am J Ophthalmol 2001;131:387–388.

2 Kadonosono K, Itoh N, Uchio E, Nakamura S, Ohno S: Staining of internal limiting membrane in macular hole surgery. Arch Ophthalmol 2000;118: 1116–1118.

3 Grizzard WS, Tornambe PE: Indocyanine green used as a vital dye to assist in the identification and removal of surface retinal membranes (video presentation). 22nd Meeting Club Jules Gonin, Taormina, 2000, p 133.

4 Haritoglou C, Gandorfer A, Kampik A: Indocyanine green can distinguish posterior vitreous cortex from internal-limiting membrane during vitrectomy with removal of epiretinal membrane. Retina 2003;23:262.

5 Gandorfer A, Haritoglou C, Gass CA, Ulbig MW, Kampik A: Indocyanine green-assisted peeling of the internal limiting membrane may cause retinal damage. Am J Ophthalmol 2001;132:431–433.

6 Gass CA, Haritoglou C, Schaumberger M, Kampik A: Functional outcome of macular hole surgery with and without indocyanine green-assisted peeling of the internal limiting membrane. Graefes Arch Clin Exp Ophthalmol 2003;241:716–720.

7 Haritoglou C, Gandorfer A, Gass CA, Schaumberger M, Ulbig MW, Kampik A: Indocyanine green-assisted peeling of the internal limiting membrane in macular hole surgery affects visual outcome: a clinicopathologic correlation. Am J Ophthalmol 2002; 134:836–841.

8 Haritoglou C, Gandorfer A, Gass CA, Kampik A: Ultrastructure of epiretinal tissue removed during indocyanine green assisted peeling in macular pucker surgery (ARVO abstract No 3516). Invest Ophthalmol Vis Sci 2002.

9 Haritoglou C, Gandorfer A, Gass CA, Schaumberger M, Ulbig MW, Kampik A: The effect of indocyanine-green on functional outcome of macular pucker surgery. Am J Ophthalmol 2003;135:328–337.

10 Haritoglou C, Gass CA, Schaumberger M, Ehrt O, Gandorfer A, Kampik A: Macular changes after peeling of the internal limiting membrane in macular hole surgery. Am J Ophthalmol 2001;132:363–368.

11 Messmer EM, Heidenkummer HP, Kampik A: Ultrastructure of epiretinal membranes associated with macular holes. Graefes Arch Clin Exp Ophthalmol 1998;236:248–254.

12 Haritoglou C, Reiniger IW, Schaumberger M, Gass CA, Priglinger SG, Kampik A: Five-year follow-up of macular hole surgery with peeling of the internal limiting membrane: update of a prospective study. Retina 2006;26:618–622.

13 Gandorfer A, Haritoglou C, Kampik A: Staining of the ILM in macular surgery. Br J Ophthalmol 2003; 87:1530.

14 Gandorfer A, Haritoglou C, Gandorfer A, Kampik A: Retinal damage from indocyanine green in experimental macular surgery. Invest Ophthalmol Vis Sci 2003;44:316–323.

15 Haritoglou C, Gandorfer A, Schaumberger M, Tadayoni R, Gandorfer A, Kampik A: Light-absorbing properties and osmolarity of indocyanine-green depending on concentration and solvent medium. Invest Ophthalmol Vis Sci 2003;44:2722–2729.

16 Haritoglou C, Gandorfer A, Gass CA, Kampik A: Histology of the vitreoretinal interface after staining of the internal limiting membrane using glucose 5% diluted indocyanine and infracyanine green. Am J Ophthalmol 2004;137:345–348.

17 Haritoglou C, Priglinger S, Gandorfer A, Welge-Lussen U, Kampik A: Histology of the vitreoretinal interface after indocyanine green staining of the ILM, with illumination using a halogen and xenon light source. Invest Ophthalmol Vis Sci 2005;46:1468–1472.

18 Grisanti S, Szurman P, Gelisken F, Aisenbrey S, Oficjalska-Mlynczak J, Bartz-Schmidt KU: Histological findings in experimental macular surgery with indocyanine green. Invest Ophthalmol Vis Sci 2004;45:282–286.

19 Kodjikian L, Richter T, Halberstadt M, Beby F, Flueckiger F, Boehnke M, Garweg JG: Toxic effects of indocyanine green, infracyanine green, and trypan blue on the human retinal pigmented epithelium. Graefes Arch Clin Exp Ophthalmol 2005;243: 917–925.

20 Ikagawa H, Yoneda M, Iwaki M, Isogai Z, Tsujii K, Yamazaki R, Kamiya T, Zako M: Chemical toxicity of indocyanine green damages retinal pigment epithelium. Invest Ophthalmol Vis Sci 2005;46:2531–2539.

21 Murata M, Shimizu S, Horiuchi S, Sato S: The effect of indocyanine green on cultured retinal glial cells. Retina 2005;25:75–80.

22 Jin Y, Uchida S, Yanagi Y, Aihara M, Araie M: Neurotoxic effects of trypan blue on rat retinal ganglion cells. Exp Eye Res 2005;81:395–400.

23 Narayanan R, Kenney MC, Kamjoo S, Trinh TH, Seigel GM, Resende GP, Kuppermann BD: Toxicity of indocyanine green (ICG) in combination with light on retinal pigment epithelial cells and neurosensory retinal cells. Curr Eye Res 2005;30:471–478.

24 Yam HF, Kwok AK, Chan KP, Lai TY, Chu KY, Lam DS, Pang CP: Effect of indocyanine green and illumination on gene expression in human retinal pigment epithelial cells. Invest Ophthalmol Vis Sci 2003;44:370–377.

25 Jackson TL, Vote B, Knight BC, El-Amir A, Stanford MR, Marshall J: Safety testing of infracyanine green using retinal pigment epithelium and glial cell cultures. Invest Ophthalmol Vis Sci 2004;45:3697–3703.

26 Enaida H, Sakamoto T, Hisatomi T, Goto Y, Ishibashi T: Morphological and functional damage of the retina caused by intravitreous indocyanine green in rat eyes. Graefes Arch Clin Exp Ophthalmol 2002; 240:209–213.

27 Schuettauf F, Haritoglou C, May CA, Rejdak R, Mankowska A, Freyer W, Eibl K, Zrenner E, Kampik A, Thaler S: Administration of novel dyes for intraocular surgery: an in vivo toxicity animal study. Invest Ophthalmol Vis Sci 2006;47:3573–3578.

28 Iriyama A, Uchida S, Yanagi Y, Tamaki Y, Inoue Y, Matsuura K, Kadonosono K, Araie M: Effects of indocyanine green on retinal ganglion cells. Invest Ophthalmol Vis Sci 2004;45:943–947.

29 Sato Y, Tomita H, Sugano E, Isago H, Yoshida M, Tamai M: Evaluation of indocyanine green toxicity to rat retinas. Ophthalmologica 2006;220:153–158.

30 Yip HK, Lai TY, So KF, Kwok AK: Retinal ganglion cells toxicity caused by photosensitising effects of intravitreal indocyanine green with illumination in rat eyes. Br J Ophthalmol 2006;90:99–102.

31 Maia M, Margalit E, Lakhanpal R, Tso MO, Grebe R, Torres G, Au Eong KG, Farah ME, Fujii GY, Weiland J, de Juan E Jr, D'Anna SA, Humayun MS: Effects of intravitreal indocyanine green injection in rabbits. Retina 2004;24:69–79.

32 Chao AN, Chen SN, Kuo YH: Retinal function and histologic changes following intravitreal injection of indocyanine green in a rabbit model. J Ocul Pharmacol Ther 2004;20:450–459.

33 Goldstein M, Zemel E, Loewenstein A, Perlman I: Retinal toxicity of indocyanine green in albino rabbits. Invest Ophthalmol Vis Sci 2006;47:2100–2107.

34 Kwok AK, Lai TY, Yeung CK, Yeung YS, Li WW, Chiang SW: The effects of indocyanine green and endoillumination on rabbit retina: an electroretinographic and histological study. Br J Ophthalmol 2005;89:897–900.

35 Maia M, Kellner L, de Juan E Jr, Smith R, Farah ME, Margalit E, Lakhanpal RR, Grebe L, Au Eong KG, Humayun MS: Effects of indocyanine green injection on the retinal surface and into the subretinal space in rabbits. Retina 2004;24:80–91.

36 Lee JE, Yoon TJ, Oum BS, Lee JS, Choi HY: Toxicity of indocyanine green injected into the subretinal space: subretinal toxicity of indocyanine green. Retina 2003;23:675–681.

37 Kawaji T, Hirata A, Inomata Y, Koga T, Tanihara H: Morphological damage in rabbit retina caused by subretinal injection of indocyanine green. Graefes Arch Clin Exp Ophthalmol 2004;242:158–164.

38 Gandorfer A, Rohleder M, Charteris DG, Sethi C, Kampik A, Luthert P: Staining and peeling of the internal limiting membrane in the cat eye. Curr Eye Res 2005;30:977–987.

39 Nakamura T, Murata T, Hisatomi T, Enaida H, Sassa Y, Ueno A, Sakamoto T, Ishibashi T: Ultrastructure of the vitreoretinal interface following the removal of the internal limiting membrane using indocyanine green. Curr Eye Res 2003;27:395–399.

40 Gandorfer A, Haritoglou C, Kampik A, Charteris D: Ultrastructure of the vitreoretinal interface following removal of the internal limiting membrane using indocyanine green. Curr Eye Res 2004;29:319–320.

41 Tokuda K, Tsukamoto T, Fujisawa S, Matsubara M: Evaluation of toxicity due to vital stains in isolated rat retinas. Acta Ophthalmol Scand 2004;82:189–194.

42 Saikia P, Maisch T, Kobuch K, Jackson TL, Baumler W, Szeimies RM, Gabel VP, Hillenkamp J: Safety testing of indocyanine green in an ex vivo porcine retina model. Invest Ophthalmol Vis Sci 2006;47:4998–5003.

43 Wollensak G, Spoerl E, Wirbelauer C, Pham DT: Influence of indocyanine green staining on the biomechanical strength of porcine internal limiting membrane. Ophthalmologica 2004;218:278–282.

44 Wollensak G, Spoerl E: Influence of indocyanine green staining on the biomechanical properties of porcine anterior lens capsule. Curr Eye Res 2004;29:413–417.

45 Haritoglou C, Freyer W, Priglinger SG, Kampik A: Light absorbing properties of indocyanine green (ICG) in solution and after adsorption to the retinal surface: an ex-vivo approach. Graefes Arch Clin Exp Ophthalmol 2006;244:1196–1202.

46 Da Mata AP, Burk SE, Riemann CD, Rosa RH Jr, Snyder ME, Petersen MR, Foster RE: Indocyanine green-assisted peeling of the retinal internal limiting membrane during vitrectomy surgery for macular hole repair. Ophthalmology 2001;108:1187–1192.

47 Da Mata AP, Burk SE, Foster RE, Riemann CD, Petersen MR, Nehemy MB, Augsburger JJ: Long-term follow-up of indocyanine green-assisted peeling of the retinal internal limiting membrane during vitrectomy surgery for idiopathic macular hole repair. Ophthalmology 2004;111:2246–2253.

48 Sheidow TG, Blinder KJ, Holekamp N, Joseph D, Shah G, Grand MG, Thomas MA, Bakal J, Sharma S: Outcome results in macular hole surgery: an evaluation of internal limiting membrane peeling with and without indocyanine green. Ophthalmology 2003;110:1697–1701.

49 Kwok AK, Lai TY, Man-Chan W, Woo DC: Indocyanine green assisted retinal internal limiting membrane removal in stage 3 or 4 macular hole surgery. Br J Ophthalmol 2003;87:71–74.

50 Lochhead J, Jones E, Chui D, Lake S, Karia N, Patel CK, Rosen P: Outcome of ICG-assisted ILM peel in macular hole surgery. Eye 2004;18:804–808.

51 Avci R, Kaderli B, Avci B, Simsek S, Baykara M, Kahveci Z, Gelisken O, Yucel AA: Pars plana vitrectomy and removal of the internal limiting membrane in the treatment of chronic macular oedema. Graefes Arch Clin Exp Ophthalmol 2004;242:845–852.
52 Lai CC, Wu WC, Chuang LH, Yeung L, Lee JS, Chen TL: Selective staining of the internal limiting membrane using the sequential intraoperative instillation of whole blood followed by indocyanine green dye. Am J Ophthalmol 2005;140:320–322.
53 Mavrofrides E, Smiddy WE, Kitchens JW, Salicone A, Feuer W: Indocyanine green-assisted internal limiting membrane peeling for macular holes: toxicity? Retina 2006;26:637–644.
54 Wrede J, Engler C, Dithmar S: Functional results after anatomically successful surgery for stage III/IV macular hole. Ophthalmologe 2006;103:935–939.
55 Oie Y, Emi K, Takaoka G, Ikeda T: Effect of indocyanine green staining in peeling of internal limiting membrane for retinal detachment resulting from macular hole in myopic eyes. Ophthalmology 2007;114:303–306.
56 Ben Simon GJ, Desatnik H, Alhalel A, Treister G, Moisseiev J: Retrospective analysis of vitrectomy with and without internal limiting membrane peeling for stage 3 and 4 macular hole. Ophthalmic Surg Lasers Imaging 2004;35:109–115.
57 Kwok AK, Li WW, Pang CP, Lai TY, Yam GH, Chan NR, Lam DS: Indocyanine green staining and removal of internal limiting membrane in macular hole surgery: histology and outcome. Am J Ophthalmol 2001;132:178–183.
58 Stalmans P, Parys-Vanginderdeuren R, De Vos R, Feron EJ: ICG staining of the inner limiting membrane facilitates its removal during surgery for macular holes and puckers. Bull Soc Belge Ophtalmol 2001;281:21–26.
59 Uemura A, Kanda S, Sakamoto Y, Kita H: Visual field defects after uneventful vitrectomy for epiretinal membrane with indocyanine green-assisted internal limiting membrane peeling. Am J Ophthalmol 2003;136:252–257.
60 Ando F, Yasui O, Hirose H, Ohba N: Optic nerve atrophy after vitrectomy with indocyanine green-assisted internal limiting membrane peeling in diffuse diabetic macular edema: adverse effect of ICG-assisted ILM peeling. Graefes Arch Clin Exp Ophthalmol 2004;242:995–999.
61 Cheng SN, Yang TC, Ho JD, Hwang JF, Cheng CK: Ocular toxicity of intravitreal indocyanine green. J Ocul Pharmacol Ther 2005;21:85–93.
62 Ueno S, Kondo M, Piao CH, Ikenoya K, Miyake Y, Terasaki H: Selective amplitude reduction of the PhNR after macular hole surgery: ganglion cell damage related to ICG-assisted ILM peeling and gas tamponade. Invest Ophthalmol Vis Sci 2006;47:3545–3549.
63 Lai TY, Kwok AK, Au AW, Lam DS: Assessment of macular function by multifocal electroretinography following epiretinal membrane surgery with indocyanine green-assisted internal limiting membrane peeling. Graefes Arch Clin Exp Ophthalmol 2007;245:148–154.
64 Engelbrecht NE, Freeman J, Sternberg P Jr, Aaberg TM Sr, Aaberg TM Jr, Martin DF, Sippy BD: Retinal pigment epithelial changes after macular hole surgery with indocyanine green-assisted internal limiting membrane peeling. Am J Ophthalmol 2002;133:89–94.
65 Wolf S, Reichel MB, Wiedemann P, Schnurrbusch UE: Clinical findings in macular hole surgery with indocyanine green-assisted peeling of the internal limiting membrane. Graefes Arch Clin Exp Ophthalmol 2003;241:589–592.
66 Posselt D, Rahman R, Smith M, Simcock PR: Visual outcomes following ICG assisted ILM peel for macular hole. Eye 2005;19:279–283.
67 Tognetto D, Haritoglou C, Kampik A, Ravalico G: Macular edema and visual loss after macular pucker surgery with ICG-assisted internal limiting membrane peeling. Eur J Ophthalmol 2005;15:289–291.
68 Sekiryu T, Iida T: Long-term observation of fundus infrared fluorescence after indocyanine green-assisted vitrectomy. Retina 2007;27:190–197.
69 Weinberger AW, Kirchhof B, Mazinani BE, Schrage NF: Persistent indocyanine green (ICG) fluorescence 6 weeks after intraocular ICG administration for macular hole surgery. Graefes Arch Clin Exp Ophthalmol 2001;239:388–390.
70 Tadayoni R, Paques M, Girmens JF, Massin P, Gaudric A: Persistence of fundus fluorescence after use of indocyanine green for macular surgery. Ophthalmology 2003;110:604–608.
71 Paques M, Genevois O, Regnier A, Tadayoni R, Sercombe R, Gaudric A, Vicaut E: Axon-tracing properties of indocyanine green. Arch Ophthalmol 2003;121:367–370.

Arnd Gandorfer, MD
Department of Ophthalmology, Ludwig-Maximilians-University
Mathildenstrasse 8
DE–80336 Munich (Germany)
Tel. +49 89 5160 3800, Fax +49 89 5160 4778, E-Mail arnd.gandorfer@med.uni-muenchen.de

Meyer CH (ed): Vital Dyes in Vitreoretinal Surgery.
Dev Ophthalmol. Basel, Karger, 2008, vol 42, pp 82–90

Biomechanical Changes of the Internal Limiting Membrane after Indocyanine Green Staining

Gregor Wollensak

Department of Ophthalmology, Vivantes-Klinikum Neukölln, Berlin, Germany

Abstract

Selective indocyanine green (ICG) staining of the macula has recently become popular in internal limiting membrane (ILM) peeling allowing a better distinction of the ILM from the underlying retina. Clinically, the ILM seems to become stiffer after ICG staining facilitating ILM peeling for the retinal surgeon. In the present study, we tried to verify the cause of this biomechanical effect. Retinal samples of postmortem porcine eyes were treated with ICG and light and compared to samples treated in darkness using biomechanical force and elongation measurements. After ICG staining of the retina combined with a 3-min illumination, a significant increase in ultimate force by 45% and a decrease in ultimate elongation by 24% were found indicating greater stiffness of the ICG-stained ILM. Without light exposure there was no such effect suggesting a light-dependent process. The stiffening effect of ICG and light is due to a photosensitizing effect of ICG leading to collagen cross-linking of the ILM.

The internal limiting membrane (ILM) is the basement membrane that forms the vitreoretinal interface and is about 2.5 μm thick. For its better visualization, indocyanine green (ICG) has become popular as a selective stain of the ILM of the retina to facilitate its surgical removal in macular disorders like cystoid edema, macular holes or pucker [1–3]. The hydrophilic dye ICG is an anionic tricarbocyanine. It does not leak into the vitreous because of its high molecular weight.

For staining the ILM, ICG solution is gently injected over the macula where it is usually left in place for about 3 min. A small slit is made in the ILM inside the vascular arcades and with the improved visibility of the stained ILM it can be relatively easily peeled off and separated from the sensory retina with a forceps. A continuous curvilinear tear is created within the vascular arcades similar to the technique applied for opening the anterior lens capsule in cataract surgery using the continuous curvilinear

This article is dedicated to Prof. Kroll for his great merits in retinal surgery.

capsulorhexis technique. After removal of the ILM, a 'negative' staining effect can be observed with the denuded area appearing unstained [1–3].

Applying ICG for ILM staining, we had the clinical impression that the ILM became somehow harder and stiffer after ICG staining, facilitating peeling also from a biomechanical aspect, similar to the lens capsule after ICG staining [4]. Therefore, we tried to systematically investigate in vitro whether ICG staining has an effect on the biomechanical properties of porcine ILM and what the cause for such changes is [5]. As the ILM could not be peeled from the postmortem porcine retina in sufficiently large sheets, we used full-thickness retina to examine the biomechanical effect.

Materials and Methods

Preparation of Specimens

The retinal specimens were prepared from a total of 40 porcine eyes from the local abattoir within 6 h after death. After sectioning the eyeball 2 mm behind the equator, the vitreous was carefully removed from the posterior segment which was turned inside out with the help of a forefinger. Using a scalpel two rectangular 10 × 7 mm retinal strips were incised in parallel above and below the plane of the optic nerve head in the temporal half of the retina and carefully transferred onto a microscope slide with the ILM side on top.

Treatment Groups

The retinal specimens were divided into the following treatment groups with always a match of one treated and one untreated control strip from the same globe:

(1) 3 min ICG staining in darkness (n = 10)
(2) 3 min white light (n = 10)
(3) 3 min ICG staining plus white light (n = 10)
(4) 30 min 0.1% glutaraldehyde (n = 10)

ICG Staining

During vitrectomy the injection of 0.2 ml of 0.05% ICG into 4 ml vitreous results in a 0.005% ICG solution (from Pulsion; Medical Systems, Munich, Germany), which was therefore chosen as the minimum ICG concentration. ICG staining was performed by dropping the 0.005% dye solution on the specimen so that the retinal strip was covered with a thin film of ICG solution. The slides were rinsed with physiologic saline solution after the intended illumination time period of 3 min.

Light Source and Spectrophotometry

External illumination was performed from a 3-cm distance using a cold-light source with an attached fiber-optic lamp (MLW, Medizinische Geräte, Berlin, Germany). The lamp had an integrated

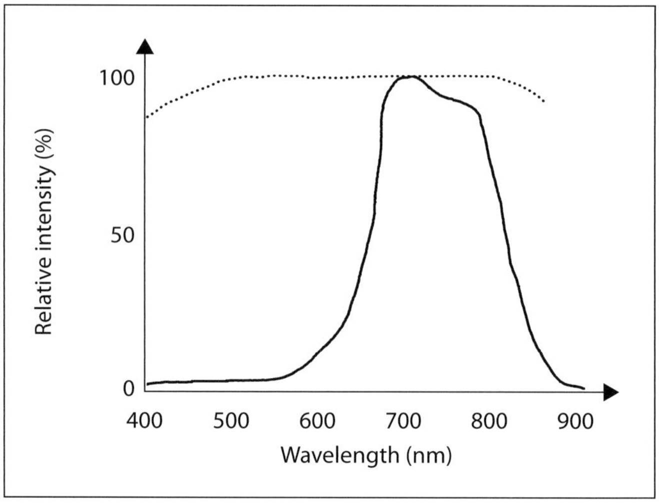

Fig. 1. Schematic drawing of the absorbance spectrum of 0.005% ICG and the emission curve (dashed line) of the cold-light source with wavelength (nm) plotted versus relative intensity (%).

infrared filter. The irradiation power was set at 6,000 lx, which was controlled with the help of a digital illumination meter (Conrad Electronics, Hirschau, Germany). The absorption spectrum of 0.005% ICG solution and the emission spectrum of the white-light fiber-optic lamp (fig. 1) were measured by a spectrophotometer (Perkins-Elmer).

Thickness Measurements

The retinal thickness was measured in histological periodic-acid-Schiff-stained sections of 5 porcine eyes.

Biomechanical Measurements

For the measurements, the retinal strips were cautiously transferred to a biomaterial test machine (Minimat, Rheometric Scientific GmbH, Bensheim, Germany) on a small piece of attached paper to facilitate the transfer. The samples were clamped horizontally between the jaws of the step-motor-driven microcomputer-controlled biomaterial tester (Minimat) with an initial distance of 4 mm (fig. 2). After the fixation of the specimens, the underlying paper was cautiously cut without damaging the specimen. A preforce of 5 mN was chosen. After that, the specimens were elongated linearly with a velocity of $2\,mm \cdot min^{-1}$. The ultimate force and ultimate elongation were measured at the tearing point (figs. 3, 4).

Statistical Evaluation

The ultimate force and elongation values at the tearing point were statistically compared between treated and untreated retinal specimens using Student's t test for paired samples.

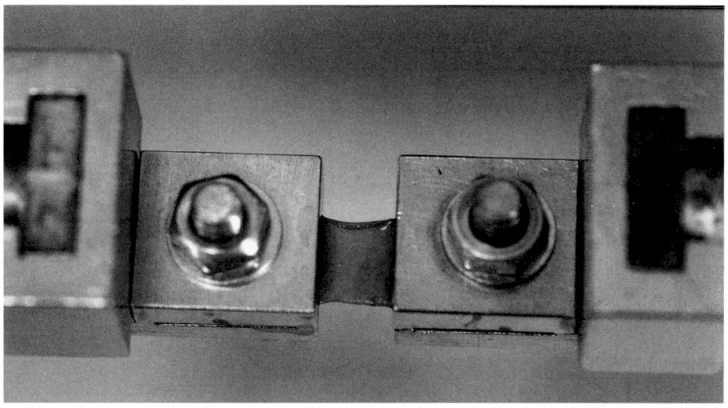

Fig. 2. Material tester (Minimat) with an ICG-stained sample of central porcine retina between the clamps.

Results

Retinal Thickness

The mean thickness of the full-thickness retina was determined histologically to be 374 ± 40 μm.

Measurements of Ultimate Force

In the specimens treated with ICG and 3 min of illumination, the ultimate force was 22.8 ± 7.5 mN compared to 15.7 ± 3.8 mN in the control retinas corresponding to an increase by 45.2% (p = 0.038). In the glutaraldehyde group, the ultimate force was 32.6 ± 9.8 mN corresponding to an increase by 107.6% (p = 0.0148).

In the specimens treated with ICG in darkness for 3 min, the ultimate force was 16.4 ± 2.8 mN (n.s., p = 0.779). In the specimens treated with light only for 3 min, the ultimate force was 15.3 ± 4.7 mN (n.s., p = 0.631) (fig. 3).

Measurements of Ultimate Elongation

In the specimens treated with ICG and light for 3 min, the ultimate elongation was 3.4 ± 0.9 mm compared to 4.5 ± 0.4 mm in the control retinas corresponding to an decrease by 24% (p = 0.015). In the glutaraldehyde group, the ultimate elongation was 1.5 ± 0.9 mm corresponding to a decrease by 66.6% (p = 0.001).

In the specimens treated with ICG in darkness, the ultimate elongation was 4.3 ± 0.3 mm (n.s., p = 0.623). In the specimens treated with light only, the ultimate elongation was 4.6 ± 0.4 mm (n.s., p = 0.582) (fig. 4).

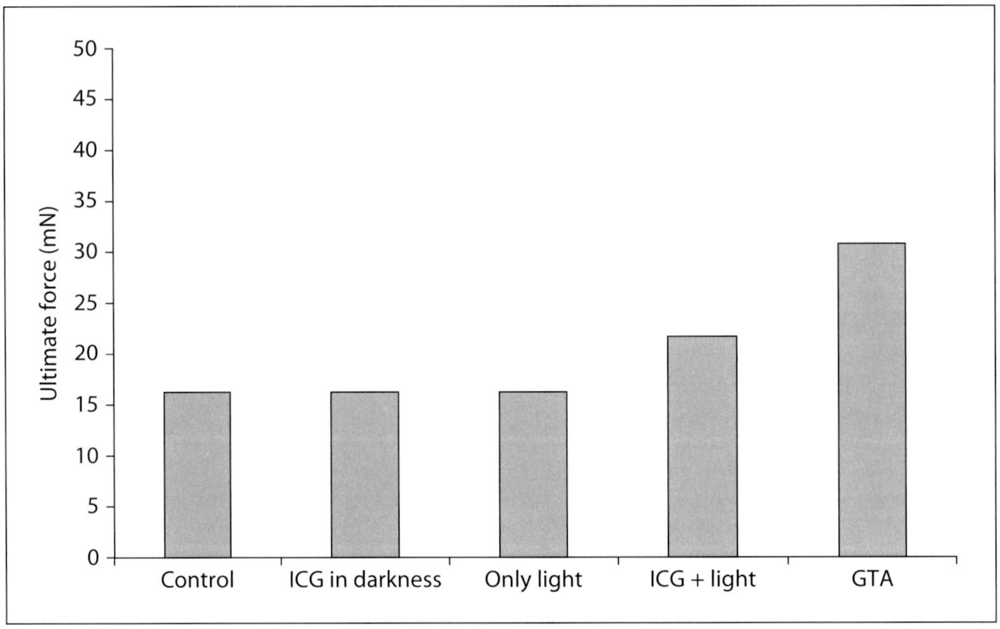

Fig. 3. Column diagram of the ultimate force (mN) at the tearing point for the different retinal treatment groups.

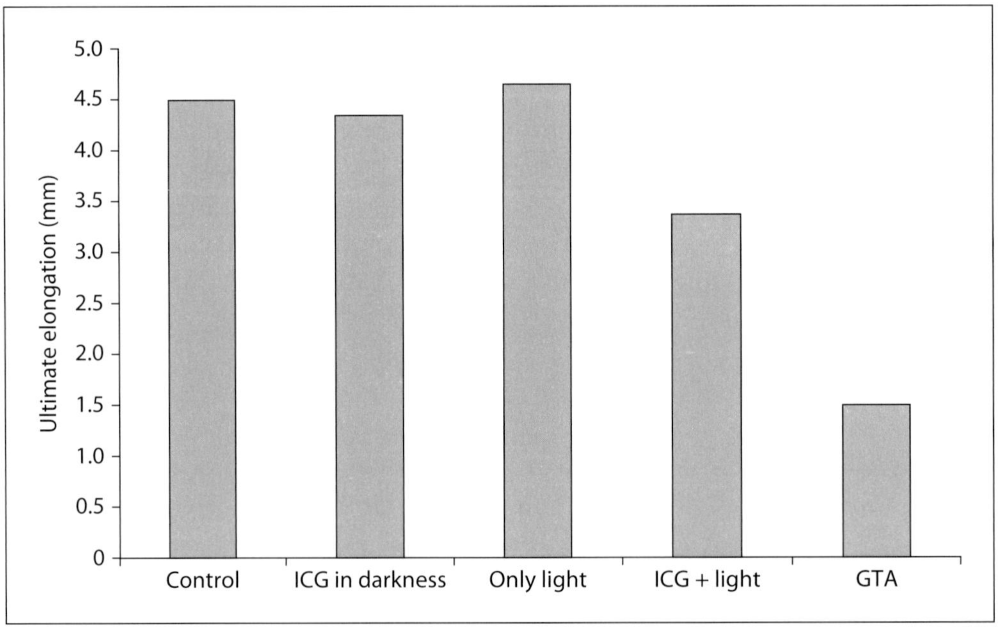

Fig. 4. Column diagram of the ultimate elongation (mm) at the tearing point for the various retinal treatment groups.

Spectrophotometry

The emission spectrum of the fiber-optic lamp was characterized by a continuous emission between 400 and 800 nm including the maximum peak of the absorption spectrum of 0.005% ICG at 700 nm [6].

Discussion

After ICG staining of the porcine retina combined with a 3-min illumination, a significant increase in ultimate force by 45% and a decrease in ultimate elongation by 24% was observed indicating an increased firmness and a reduced elasticity of the stained ILM.

Remarkably, there was no such stiffening effect after ICG staining in the darkness indicating a light-dependent process. In fact, ICG is known to be a photosensitizer from other studies [7]. The first step in the photodynamic process is the absorption of light by the photosensitizer ICG which produces an excited state of the ICG molecule, the so-called triplet state, creating reactive oxygen species like superoxide anion O_2^-, hydrogen peroxide H_2O_2, and hydroxyl radical HO^-, mainly in the so-called type I reaction of photooxidation (fig. 5) [8]. The reactive oxygen species in turn lead to photooxidative damage of cells and physical cross-linking of collagen which are both two sides of the same coin so to speak [9].

Correspondingly, recent studies have also shown a photooxidative toxic effect of ICG in its use for dye-enhanced ILM peeling with cellular damage in the superficial ganglion cells of the retina similar to a 'sunburn' that damages the external skin [1, 3, 5]. The photooxidative damage due to ICG-potentiated light toxicity could be prevented by using a filter that blocks the wavelengths of the light source beyond 620 nm being critical for the ICG absorption, which reveals the great relevance of the photosensitizing effect of ICG [5]. In addition, the light pipe should be kept far from the retina to minimize the ICG-mediated photosensitizer effects [1]. Other possible critical factors of ICG staining are the osmolarity of the ICG solution, direct toxicity by ICG itself and an abnormal cleavage plane and therefore damage to the innermost retinal layers [1, 3].

It is not surprising that glutaraldehyde, which is a very efficient chemical cross-linker [10] of collagen, induced the highest increase in the biomechanical stiffness demonstrated by an increase in ultimate force by 107% and a decrease in ultimate elongation by 66.6%.

Our measurements were only performed on full-thickness retina and not on isolated ILM specimens because it was not possible to prepare large enough intact sheets of ILM. However, the use of the full-thickness retina in our measurements is corroborated by the fact that after ICG staining the ILM is stained selectively without the underlying retinal layers [1, 2] so that photosensitized cross-linking should also

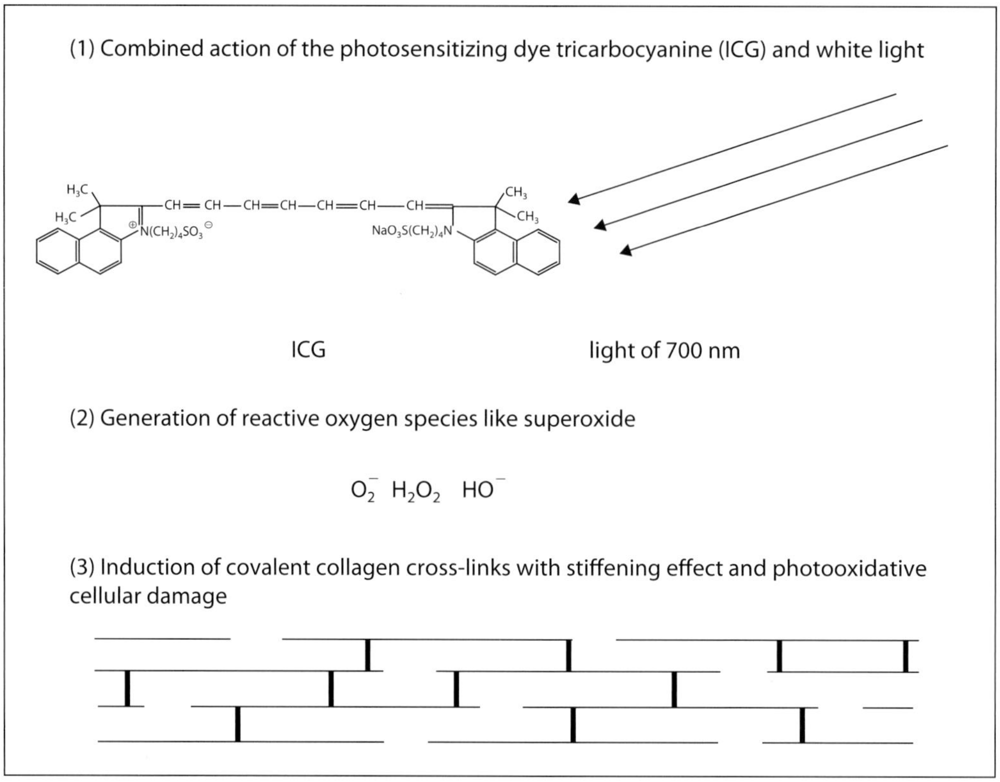

Fig. 5. Scheme of the photodynamic action of ICG combined with white-light irradiation leading to cross-linking of the ILM.

occur only in the ILM. Similarly, phototoxic damage after ICG staining was only found in the ILM and the immediately adjacent nerve fiber layer and ganglion cells [1, 3, 5] and not in the deeper retinal layers.

The biomechanical observations of the present study also underline the clinical significance of biomechanical findings of the ILM and retina [11, 12], which have been scarcely considered so far by retinal surgeons. So for example, it has been shown that the retina has a tearing point 170 times lower than the choroid predisposing to retinal tears but also an ability for plastic irreversible deformation protecting against tears [11]. As for the ILM, it has been demonstrated that the ILM of the posterior pole contributes significantly to the biomechanical stability of the retina because after removal of the ILM the mean force of the retina was reduced by 53.6% [12].

So far there have been no reports on cross-linking of the ILM as a natural phenomenon. However, analogous cross-linking-related biomechanical changes have been observed for the lens capsule with glycation-induced cross-linking in diabetes mellitus [13], cross-linking due to aging [14] and after staining with ICG or trypan blue [3, 15]. These reports on cross-linking of the lens capsule under various conditions are also relevant for the ILM because the lens capsule and the ILM are comparable periodic-acid-Schiff-positive basement membranes both made up of a network of collagen type IV and proteoglycans [16]. Interestingly, cross-linkage of proteins also is the main cause for cataract formation leading to hardening and opacification of the lens [17].

The increased elastic stiffness and greater firmness of the ILM after ICG-induced cross-linking should facilitate the surgical procedure and control of the continuous curvilinear tear in ILM peeling allowing a better grip of the ILM and a smoother rim of the ILM rhexis. Similarly, the young lens capsule is significantly more elastic than the more cross-linked and stiffer adult lens capsule, making the continuous curvilinear capsulorhexis of the lens capsule more challenging [18].

In summary, ICG staining combined with illumination for 3 min leads to a significant increase in the biomechanical strength and a decrease in elasticity of the porcine ILM due to photosensitizer-mediated collagen cross-linking of the ILM. This is another advantage of ICG staining in addition to the effect of a better visualization of the ILM.

References

1 Rodrigues EB, Meyer CH, Farah ME, Kroll P: Intravitreal staining of the internal limiting membrane using indocyanine green in the treatment of macular holes. Ophthalmologica 2005;219: 251–262.

2 Gandorfer A, Messmer EM, Ulbig MW, Kampik A: Indocyanine green selectively stains the internal limiting membrane. Am J Ophthalmol 2001;131: 387–388.

3 Gandorfer A, Haritoglou C, Gass CA, Ulbig MW, Kampik A: Indocyanine green-assisted peeling of the internal limiting membrane may cause retinal damage. Am J Ophthalmol 2001;132:431–433.

4 Wollensak G, Spoerl E: Influence of indocyanine green staining on the biomechanical properties of porcine anterior lens capsule. Curr Eye Res 2004; 29:413–417.

5 Wollensak G, Spoerl E, Wirbelauer C, Pham D-T: Influence of indocyanine green staining on the biomechanical strength of porcine internal limiting membrane. Ophthalmologica 2004;218:278–282.

6 Gandorfer A, Haritoglou C, Gandorfer A, Kampik A: Retinal damage from indocyanine green in experimental macular surgery. Invest Ophthalmol Vis Sci 2003;44:316–323.

7 Costa RA, Farah ME, Freymüller E, Morales PH, Smith R, Cardillo J: Choriocapillaris photodynamic therapy using indocyanine green. Am J Ophthalmol 2002;132:557–565.

8 Foote CS: Definition of type I and type II photosensitized oxidation. Photochem Photobiol 1991;54: 659.

9 Andley U: Photooxidative stress; in Albert DM, Jakobiec F (eds): Principles and Practice of Ophthalmology. Philadelphia, WB Saunders Co, 1992, vol 1, pp 575–590.

10 Charulatha V, Rajaram A: Influence of different crosslinking treatments on the physical properties of collagen membranes. Biomaterials 2003;24: 759–767.

11 Wollensak G, Spoerl E: Biomechanical characteristics of retina. Retina 2004;24:967–970.

12 Wollensak G, Spoerl E, Grosse G, Wirbelauer C: Biomechanical significance of the human internal limiting lamina. Retina 2006;26:965–968.

13 Bailey AJ, Sims TJ, Avery NC, Miles CA: Chemistry of collagen cross-links: glucose-mediated covalent cross-linking of type-IV collagen in lens capsules. Biochem J 1993;296:489–496.

14 Krag S, Olsen T, Andreassen TT: Biomechanical characteristics of the human anterior lens capsule in relation to age. Invest Ophthalmol Vis Sci 1997;38: 357–363.
15 Wollensak G, Spörl E, Pham D-T: Biomechanical changes in the anterior lens capsule after trypan blue staining. J Cataract Refract Surg 2004;30: 1526–1530.
16 Johan PS, Spiro RG: Macromolecular organization of basement membranes. J Biol Chem 1986;261: 4328–4336.
17 Bellows JG, Bellows RT: Crosslinkage theory of senile cataracts. Ann Ophthalmol 1976;8:129–135.
18 Auffarth GU, Wesendahl TA, Newland TJ, Apple DJ: Capsulorhexis in the rabbit eye as a model for pediatric capsulectomy. J Cataract Refract Surg 1994; 20:188–191.

PD Dr. Gregor Wollensak
Wildentensteig 4
DE–14195 Berlin (Germany)
Tel. +49 30 826 4499, Fax +49 30 826 449, E-Mail gwollens@hotmail.com

Meyer CH (ed): Vital Dyes in Vitreoretinal Surgery.
Dev Ophthalmol. Basel, Karger, 2008, vol 42, pp 91–100

Current Concepts of Trypan Blue in Chromovitrectomy

Michel E. Farah · Mauricio Maia · Bruno Furlani · Juliana Bottós · Carsten H. Meyer · Veronica Lima · Fernando M. Penha · Elaine F. Costa · Eduardo B. Rodrigues

Vision Institute, Department of Ophthalmology, Federal University of Sao Paulo, Sao Paulo, Brazil

Abstract

Trypan blue (TB) is a blue vital dye with fine color properties to stain the anterior lens capsule and thereby may facilitate capsulorrhexis during cataract surgery. In addition, the blue stain may assist in the visualization of various preretinal membranes and tissues during vitreoretinal surgery in a procedure also called chromovitrectomy. TB has demonstrated great binding affinity for the glial epiretinal membranes, although it remains yet to be determined in which circumstances the dye may color the vitreous and internal limiting membrane. Most studies suggest that 0.06% TB does not pose harm to the retina, but at higher concentrations further investigation is necessary. In this paper, various aspects of the application of TB for chromovitrectomy are discussed including laboratory investigations, surgical technique and clinical outcomes.

Trypan blue (TB) is a vital stain which has been widely used in ocular surgery. Since the end of the 1990s, the blue dye has demonstrated great affinity properties for the anterior lens capsule and thereby facilitated capsulorrhexis for cataract surgery [1]. Soon thereafter, vitreoretinal surgeons noted the success of cataract surgeons using vital stains, and started the intraoperative application of vital dyes to identify preretinal membranes and tissues. Indeed, TB dye promoted staining of the acellular internal limiting membrane (ILM) and the glial epiretinal membrane (ERM) in chromovitrectomy [2, 3]. Concomitantly, numerous publications reported in vitro and in vivo toxicity of TB to various retinal cellular elements [4–6]. In this paper, an overview of the application of TB in ocular and vitreoretinal surgery in recent years is presented.

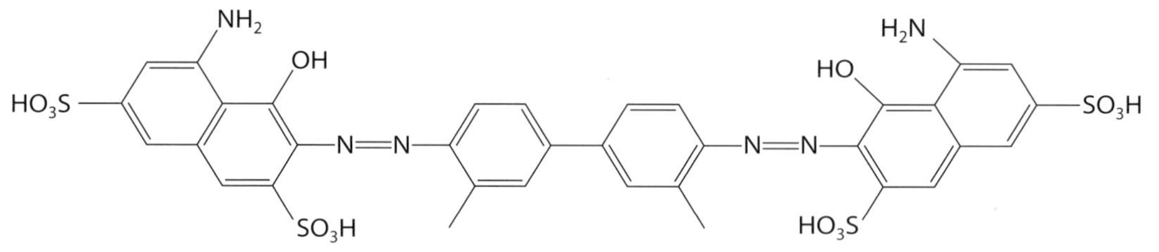

Fig. 1. Chemical structure of TB. TB is derived from toluidine with several isomeric bases and the formula of $C_{34}H_{24}N_6Na_4O_{14}S_4$.

Physicochemical Properties of Trypan Blue

TB was first synthesized by the German scientist Paul Ehrlich in 1904, and received this name because it can kill trypanosomes. In chemistry, TB belongs to the anionic diazo type of vital dyes with the chemical formula $C_{34}H_{24}N_6Na_4O_{14}S_4$ and a molecular weight of 960 Da (fig. 1). The large water-soluble blue dye has also been called diamine blue and Niagara blue. Live cells or tissues with intact cell membranes are not colored with TB because the cell membranes in living cells do not allow passage or absorption of the blue dye; however, TB traverses the membrane in a dead cell. Hence, dead cells are shown in a distinctive blue color under a microscope. This is a well-known staining method called dye exclusion method. The blue dye absorbs light at around 580 nm, which may overlap with current vitrectomy probes (fig. 2).

The Use and Safety of Trypan Blue in Biology, Medicine, and Ophthalmic Surgery

TB has frequently been used in microscopy for cell counting for staining of the reticuloendothelial system and the kidney tubules. In ocular surgery, TB has initially been applied to evaluate the endothelial viability of the donor cornea just prior to keratoplasty. The blue dye enabled recognition of the viability of the endothelial cells, which indicate the quality of the donor corneal endothelium, an important factor for the successful outcome of penetrating keratoplasty [7]. More recently, TB has been recognized as a useful adjuvant for recognition of the anterior capsule during cataract surgery when the red reflex for the capsulorrhexis maneuver is not possible [1]. For ocular surgery, TB is available in the concentration of 0.06 or 0.15%. The Ophthalmic Technology Assessment Committee Anterior Segment Panel of the American Academy of Ophthalmology published an analysis of the literature on capsular staining

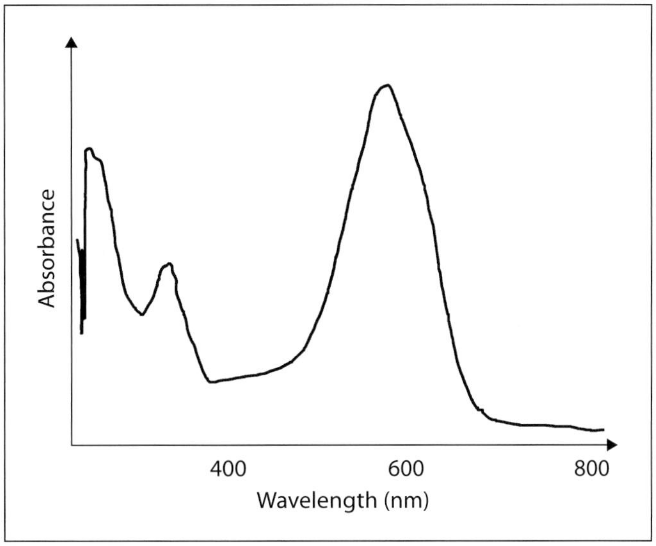

Fig. 2. Absorbance versus wavelength curve of TB diluted in balanced salt solution. The dye shows a peak absorbance of 380 λ at 580 nm.

for cataract surgery in 2006. They reported level III evidence (case series and case reports) that TB is both easy to use and visualize the anterior capsule; in addition, they found substantial data on the safety of using TB in the anterior chamber [8].

Various theories and evidence have arisen in regard to the toxic effects of TB on human tissues. In 1971, Vlckova et al. [9] postulated that the two main color components of TB, monoazo and bisazo, might be responsible for its toxicity. However, they could not exclude the chance that impurities present in the commercial products might be responsible for the harmful properties. According to further experiments systemic TB has been shown to promote carcinogenic and mutagenic cellular effects [10].

Surgical Application of Trypan Blue in Chromovitrectomy

There are four main target tissues for TB staining during chromovitrectomy.

(a) ERMs: TB exhibits outstanding affinity for ERMs because of the strong presence of dead glial cells within those membranes. Various investigators, including our group, agree that the state-of-the-art vitrectomy mandates TB application for recognition of ERMs of various etiologies, as the blue dye enables complete identification of the entire ERM surface [11, 12]. Nonetheless, the exact dose of TB necessary for ERM staining remains yet to be determined.

(b) ILM: few clinical reports have advocated the use of TB to stain the acellular ILM and facilitate its removal [13, 14]. However, ILM staining with TB is subtler than

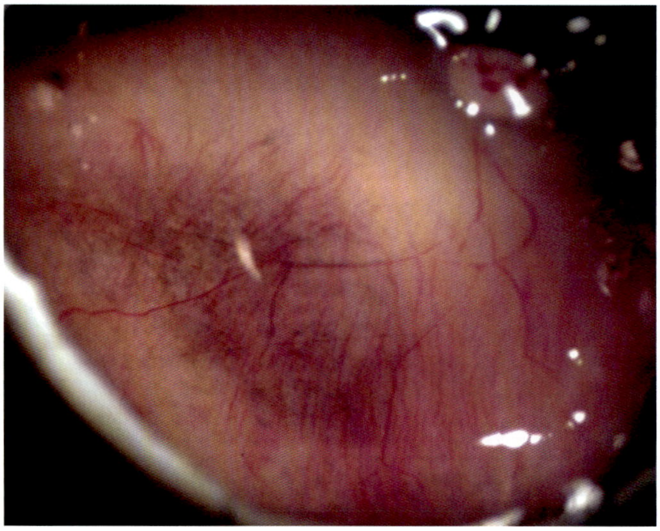

Fig. 3. The blue dye TB in animal experiments in enucleated porcine eyes promoted only faint ILM staining.

with the vital dye indocyanine green (ICG), and possibly TB rather stains the fine ERM overlying the ILM but not the ILM itself (fig. 3).

(c) Vitreous: the usefulness of intracameral or intravitreal injection of TB to highlight vitreous gel has recently been proposed. The blue dye in various doses may enable the visualization of both prolapsed vitreous to the anterior chamber or posterior vitreous remaining in the vitreous cavity [15, 16]. However, TB application for vitreous visualization has not gained much popularity because newer vital dyes, for example triamcinolone, may stain the vitreous better than TB.

(d) Retinal breaks: a new application for TB in chromovitrectomy consists in staining retinal break edges during vitrectomy for rhegmatogenous retinal detachment repair. TB 0.15% has been injected transretinally into the subretinal space using a 41-gauge cannula designed for macular translocation surgery. Jackson et al. [17] demonstrated the success of this technique to identify retinal breaks in 4 out of 5 patients and concluded TB-guided retinal break detection to be a very useful surgical technique.

Substantial surgical experience in most studies in recent years revealed that TB application promotes positive anatomical and visual outcomes in chromovitrectomy. TB staining during vitrectomy induced no significant intra- or postoperative signs of toxicity. In addition, it allowed complete removal of ERMs of various causes and of the ILM during macular hole surgery. Moreover, it induced vision stabilization or improvement [3, 11, 13, 14, 18–20]. Haritoglou et al. [19] investigated functional outcomes of macular pucker surgery with and without the use of 0.15% TB for a mean follow-up time of 4–6 months in 20 patients. Postoperatively, the median visual acuity difference between the two groups was not statistically significant; however, 4 of 10 patients without and 7 of 10 patients with TB staining experienced an improvement of visual acuity of 2 lines or more. Two published studies evaluated the anatomical and visual outcomes after vitrectomy and ILM peeling for idiopathic macular hole repair in patients with stage II–IV idiopathic macular holes using ICG or TB. The rate of macular hole closures was the same; however, visual recovery was significant only in the TB group [14, 21]. A similar comparison between TB and ICG for ERM removal also indicated encouraging results with the blue dye injection. All eyes had symptomatic improvement, none developed ERM recurrence, and no complication related to TB or ICG was observed clinically or angiographically [22].

In contrast to the reported safe clinical outcomes using TB in chromovitrectomy, some investigations with histology examination disclosed that TB staining may exert some amount of retinal damage especially at higher concentrations. Veckeneer et al. [6] showed striking retinal alterations including disintegration of retinal architecture and photoreceptor destruction in the eyes injected with 0.2% TB. Gandorfer et al. [23] examined the feline as a model for TB- and ICG-guided peeling of the ILM; TB staining promoted no ultrastructural retinal damage, but there were fragments of Müller cells adherent to the retinal side of the ILM, and Müller cell end feet were ruptured and avulsed. Finally, one recent report released in 2004 disclosed that electron microscopy of TB-stained ERM specimens showed fragments of the ILM in all specimens [22]. The clinical relevance of those ultrastructural findings remains to be determined; however, future controlled studies should clarify whether or not TB use may be clinically toxic at all.

Laboratory Experiments to Evaluate Retinal Toxicity of Intravitreal Trypan Blue

In vitro Experiments for Evaluation of Trypan Blue Toxicity

In vitro experiments use a controlled setting for the investigation of a clinically relevant question. For in vitro evaluation of retinal toxicity, both the epithelial type of cell, i.e. retinal pigment epithelial (RPE) cells, and the neuroretinal cells may be examined after exposure to various drugs and chemicals. The toxic effects of TB on neuroretinal cells have been investigated by some investigators in recent years. Both Narayanan et al. [4] and Jin et al. [24] observed a dose-dependent damage to rodent neurosensory cells in vitro after TB exposure at various concentrations ranging from 0.0125 to 0.1%. Narayanan et al. [4] noticed that neuroretinal cells were in general very sensible to TB exposure at all concentrations. In addition, they also found a stronger toxicity of TB at higher doses and with light exposure using the mitochondrial dehydrogenase assay [4]. In the second study, TB promoted toxic effects on cultured retinal ganglion cells in a time- and dose-dependent manner, suggesting that TB may induce significant neuroretinal damage after an exposure time longer than 2 min [24]. In contrast to those results, one study with cell culture investigation demonstrated no cellular damage after TB exposure to glial cells at concentrations of up to 0.2% [25]. Additional investigations should elucidate the reason for the more likely damage of glial cells in comparison to retinal ganglion cells. To decrease the risk of neuroretinal damage by TB during chromovitrectomy, surgeons should expose retinal tissue to a low TB concentration and short period of time.

A substantial amount of in vitro experiments proposed that TB may be safe to RPE cells. Narayanan et al. [4] examined the effects of TB exposure on human RPE cells called ARPE-19 and observed, using the dye exclusion method, that TB at concentrations from 0.1 to 0.0125% with or without light exposure did not affect RPE cell viability. Stalmans et al. [26] performed an in vitro study on the cell viability of cultured human RPE cells stained with TB at concentrations of 0.06, 0.15, and 0.30% using confocal microscopy. No increased cell death was found in cultures incubated with any of the TB concentrations investigated. The authors suggested that acute TB exposure of RPE cells may be safe. Some recent in vitro studies matched those previous results, since they demonstrated that TB induced no toxicity to RPE cells after acute and chronic exposure [27, 28].

On the other hand, a few researchers have found variable degrees of toxicity after TB exposure of RPE cells. Kodjikian et al. [29] evaluated the acute and chronic toxicities of TB in cultured human RPE cells using concentrations from 0.05 to 0.5% for 5 min or 6 days (chronic exposure). TB yielded no acute toxicity but it was chronically cytotoxic at all tested concentrations. Kwok et al. [30] evaluated the effects of three concentrations of TB (0.06, 0.6, and 4 mg/ml) on cell viability, apoptosis markers, and gene expression in human RPE cells. Their results showed that TB at the two higher concentrations may lead to toxicity in cultured RPE cells, as indicated by the reduction in cell viability and changes in the expression of apoptotic and cell cycle arrest genes. Another investigation analyzed if TB leads to RPE cell apoptosis in vitro in pure RPE cell cultures. The cells were incubated with different concentrations of TB of 0.5, 0.10, and 0.05% for 5 or 30 min. TB promoted a significant amount of RPE cell apoptosis at all concentrations investigated [31]. Some of the reasons for conflicting results in the literature in regard to RPE cell toxicity with TB include the difference in the concentrations of TB in each experiment, the technique for evaluation of toxicity and apoptosis assessment (Annexin V staining, cytometry), or the timing of the cell viability measurement (chronic or acute).

Hirasawa et al. [32], in 2007, investigated whether TB may be taken up by RPE cells, and found that the blue dye was not taken up by RPE cells in their experimental settings. This might be because TB is membrane impermeable and will not be incorporated into the cells. Therefore, it may be possible to remove TB almost completely after chromovitrectomy, suggesting that extensive wash after ILM staining is a key procedure to minimize residual dye in the vitreous cavity and ocular tissues.

In vivo Animal Experiments for Evaluation of Trypan Blue Toxicity

Various animal experiments disclosed opposite results regarding retinal toxicity of TB, while some studies of rabbit and rat eyes demonstrated dose-dependent retinal toxicity of TB. Veckeneer et al. [6] reported the lack of both histological and electrophysiological retinal toxicity in rabbit eyes 4 weeks after intravitreal injection of 0.06% TB. However, at a higher concentration of 0.2% TB, light and electron microscopy revealed damaged photoreceptors and marked retinal layer disorganization in the inferior retina. In another study, TB at a concentration of 0.02% was found to be safe but there was disorganization of the inner retinal layers at concentrations of 0.15 and 0.25% [19]. Luce et al. [33] investigated the effects of 0.15% TB on bovine retinal function in retinal preparations perfused with a standard solution with electroretinogram recording. The authors also revealed irreversible toxic effects of 0.15% TB after a short period of retinal exposure in a bovine model, manifested by loss of the b-wave after retinal exposure longer than 15 s. In contrast to these negative outcomes, in a recent study, Tokuda et al. [34] found no retinal harm after intravitreal low-dose TB injections of rat retina tissue using morphologic examination and lactate dehydrogenase assay. The contradictions between the two studies may be explained by differences in methodology; for instance, some surgeons performed intravitreal injections of TB which enabled the dilution of the dye inside the vitreous cavity of the rabbit eyes before retinal contact, while others applied the blue dye directly onto the retinal surface. Nevertheless, these findings in general suggest that TB at lower concentrations of 0.02–0.06% may be used in vitreoretinal surgery.

Our research group has recently conducted two investigation projects to examine the influence of subretinal injections of TB and other dyes in rabbits. In a first series of experiments, we evaluated the effects of subretinal injections of 0.5% ICG, 0.15% TB, glucose, and balanced salt solution (BSS) in rabbits. Animals were examined 6, 12, and 24 h and 14 days after the procedure by fluorescein angiography and fundus evaluation. Histologic studies were performed by light and transmission electron microscopy. Fluorescein angiography showed window defects where ICG and TB had been injected. Subretinal injection of TB resulted in histologic abnormalities 24 h and 14 days after surgery. Hypoosmolar TB caused edema of the photoreceptor outer segments (POS) and the photoreceptor inner segments (PIS) and pyknosis of the outer nuclear layer (ONL) 6 and 12 h after surgery. The RPE was also affected 24 h and 14 days after surgery. The damage induced by hypoosmolar solutions was more important than that caused by the isoosmolar colored and noncolored solutions [35]. In a second project, we compared the angiographic and histologic effects of subretinal 0.15% TB with those of 0.24% Prussian blue (PB) and BSS in rabbits. Our studies revealed window defects using fluorescent antibody examination suggestive of RPE atrophy in positions of subretinal TB injection, which was not observed following subretinal injection of PB or BSS. Histological evaluation disclosed only minimal abnormalities on the POS after subretinal injection of BSS during all follow-ups. Subretinal injection of PB promoted POS and PIS abnormalities 12 and 24 h following surgery as well as ONL damage 14 days after surgery. Subretinal TB injection induced POS and PIS damage at 12 h of follow-up. The ONL damage was observed 24 h after surgery; additionally, POS, PIS, ONL and RPE abnormalities were noted 14 days following surgery after TB injection [36]. In addition to those findings, our investigation demonstrated a higher 'resistance' of RPE cells to various subretinal dyes including TB, as well as a faster subretinal reabsorption of PB compared to TB. Future human studies are necessary to evaluate the clinical relevance of these in vivo experiments.

Final Remarks

TB arose as a remarkable biostain for surgical application during chromovitrectomy. While the blue azo dye has intraoperatively demonstrated strong binding affinity for the glial ERMs, it remains yet to be determined at which concentrations the dye may be used to stain the ILM and the vitreous. Most studies agreed that 0.06% TB is safe to the retina, although at higher concentrations the risk of retinal toxicity exists. The blue dye may be diluted in glucose 5 or 10% in order to facilitate its staining by deposition onto the posterior preretinal membranes and tissues; however, higher glucose concentrations should be avoided since glucose 50% has a highly toxic osmolarity of 1,150 mosm. In the future, clinical investigations should clarify the role of TB in combination with other vital dyes, so-called double staining, and determine the safe dose of intravitreal TB for chromovitrectomy.

Acknowledgment

This work has been supported by the Fehr Foundation, Marburg, Germany, the FAPESP-Fundação de amparo a Pesquisa do Estado de Sao Paulo, and by the PAOF-Pan-American Ophthalmological Foundation.

References

1 Melles GR, de Waard PW, Pameyer JH, Houdijn Beekhuis W: Trypan blue capsule staining to visualize the capsulorhexis in cataract surgery. J Cataract Refract Surg 1999;25:7–9.

2 Rodrigues EB, Meyer CH, Kroll P: Chromovitrectomy: a new field in vitreoretinal surgery. Graefes Arch Clin Exp Ophthalmol 2005;243: 291–293.

3 Teba FA, Mohr A, Eckardt C, Wong D, Kusaka S, Joondeph BC, Feron EJ, Stalmans P, Van Overdam K, Melles GR: Trypan blue staining in vitreoretinal surgery. Ophthalmology 2003;110:2409–2412.

4 Narayanan R, Kenney MC, Kamjoo S, Trinh TH, Seigel GM, Resende GP, Kuppermann BD: Trypan blue: effect on retinal pigment epithelial and neurosensory retinal cells. Invest Ophthalmol Vis Sci 2005;46:304–309.

5 Luke C, Luke M, Sickel W, Schneider T: Effects of patent blue on human retinal function. Graefes Arch Clin Exp Ophthalmol 2006;244:1188–1190.

6 Veckeneer M, van Overdam K, Monzer J, Kobuch K, van Marle W, Spekreijse H, van Meurs J: Ocular toxicity study of trypan blue injected into the vitreous cavity of rabbit eyes. Graefes Arch Clin Exp Ophthalmol 2001;239:698–704.

7 Singh G, Böhnke M, von-Domarus D, Draeger J, Lindstrom RL, Doughman DJ: Vital staining of corneal endothelium. Cornea 1985;4:80–91.

8 Jacobs DS, Cox TA, Wagoner MD, Ariyasu RG, Karp CL, American Academy of Ophthalmology, Ophthalmic Technology Assessment Committee Anterior Segment Panel: Capsule staining as an adjunct to cataract surgery: a report from the American Academy of Ophthalmology. Ophthalmology 2006; 113:707–713.

9 Vlckova A, Gasparic J, Horakova K: Investigation of the cytotoxicity of different trypan blue commercial products. Bull Acad Pol Sci Biol 1971;19: 763–770.

10 Chung KT: The significance of azo-reduction in the mutagenesis and carcinogenesis of azo dyes. Mutat Res 1983;114:269–281.

11 Perrier M, Sébag M: Epiretinal membrane surgery assisted by trypan blue. Am J Ophthalmol 2003;135: 909–911.

12 Feron EJ, Veckeneer M, Parys-Van Ginderdeuren R, Van Lommel A, Melles GR, Stalmans P: Trypan blue staining of epiretinal membranes in proliferative vitreoretinopathy. Arch Ophthalmol 2002;120: 141–144.

13 Li K, Wong D, Hiscott P, Stanga P, Groenewald C, McGalliard J: Trypan blue staining of the internal limiting membrane and epiretinal membrane during vitrectomy: visual results and histopathological findings. Br J Ophthalmol 2003;87:216–219.

14 Lee KL, Dean S, Guest S: A comparison of outcomes after indocyanine green and trypan blue assisted internal limiting membrane peeling during macular hole surgery. Br J Ophthalmol 2005;89: 420–424.

15 Cacciatori M, Chadha V, Bennett HG, Singh J: Trypan blue to aid visualization of the vitreous during anterior segment surgery. J Cataract Refract Surg 2006;32:389–391.

16 Verma L, Prakash G, Tewari HK: Trypan blue enhanced vitrectomy in clear gel vitrectomy. Indian J Ophthalmol 2003;51:106.

17 Jackson TL, Kwan AS, Laidlaw AH, Aylward W: Identification of retinal breaks using subretinal trypan blue injection. Ophthalmology 2007;114: 587–590.

18 Balayre S, Boissonnot M, Curutchet L, Dighiero P: Role of trypan blue in epiretinal membrane surgery. J Fr Ophtalmol 2005;28:290–297.

19 Haritoglou C, Gandorfer A, Schaumberger M, Priglinger SG, Mueller AJ, Gass CA, Kampik A: Trypan blue in macular pucker surgery: an evaluation of histology and functional outcome. Retina 2004;24: 582–590.

20 Vote BJ, Russell MK, Joondeph BC: Trypan blue-assisted vitrectomy. Retina 2004;24:736–738.

21 Beutel J, Dahmen G, Ziegler A, Hoerauf H: Internal limiting membrane peeling with indocyanine green or trypan blue in macular hole surgery: a randomized trial. Arch Ophthalmol 2007;125:326–332.

22 Kwok AK, Lai TY, Li WW, Yew DT, Wong VW: Trypan blue- and indocyanine green-assisted epiretinal membrane surgery: clinical and histopathological studies. Eye 2004;18:882–888.

23 Gandorfer A, Rohleder M, Charteris DG, Sethi C, Kampik A, Luthert P: Staining and peeling of the internal limiting membrane in the cat eye. Curr Eye Res 2005;30:977–987.

24 Jin Y, Uchida S, Yanagi Y, Aihara M, Araie M: Neurotoxic effects of trypan blue on rat retinal ganglion cells. Exp Eye Res 2005;81:395–400.

25 Jackson TL, Hillenkamp J, Knight BC, Zhang JJ, Thomas D, Stanford MR, Marshall J: Safety testing of indocyanine green and trypan blue using retinal pigment epithelium and glial cell cultures. Invest Ophthalmol Vis Sci 2004;45:2778–2785.

26 Stalmans P, Van Aken EH, Melles G, Veckeneer M, Feron EJ, Stalmans I: Trypan blue not toxic for retinal pigment epithelium in vitro. Am J Ophthalmol 2003;135:234–236.

27 Gale JS, Proulx AA, Gonder JR, Mao AJ, Hutnik CM: Comparison of the in-vitro toxicity of indocyanine green to that of trypan blue in human retinal pigment epithelium cell cultures. Am J Ophthalmol 2004;138:64–69.

28 Mennel S, Thumann G, Peter S, Meyer CH, Kroll P: Influence of vital dyes on the function of the outer blood-retinal barrier in vitro. Klin Monatsbl Augenheilkd 2006;223:568–576.

29 Kodjikian L, Richter T, Halberstadt M, Beby F, Flueckiger F, Boehnke M, Garweg JG: Toxic effects of indocyanine green, infracyanine green, and trypan blue on the human retinal pigmented epithelium. Graefes Arch Clin Exp Ophthalmol 2005;243: 917–925.

30 Kwok AK, Yeung CK, Lai TY, Chan KP, Pang CP: Effects of trypan blue on cell viability and gene expression in human retinal pigment epithelial cells. Br J Ophthalmol 2004;88:1590–1594.

31 Rezai KA, Farrokh-Siar L, Gasyna EM, Ernest JT: Trypan blue induces apoptosis in human retinal pigment epithelial cells. Am J Ophthalmol 2004;138: 492–495.

32 Hirasawa H, Yanagi Y, Tamaki Y, Inoue Y, Kadonosono K: Indocyanine green and trypan blue: intracellular uptake and extracellular binding by human retinal pigment epithelial cells. Retina 2007; 27:375–378.
33 Luke C, Luke M, Dietlein TS, et al: Retinal tolerance to dyes. Br J Ophthalmol 2005;89:1188–1191.
34 Tokuda K, Tsukamoto T, Fujisawa S, Matsubara M: Evaluation of toxicity due to vital stains in isolated rat retinas. Acta Ophthalmol Scand 2004;82: 189–194.
35 Penha FM, Maia M, Eid Farah M, Príncipe AH, Freymüller EH, Maia A, Magalhães O, Smith RL: Effects of subretinal injections of indocyanine green, trypan blue, and glucose in rabbit eyes. Ophthalmology 2007;114:899–908.
36 Maia M, Penha FM, Rodrigues EB, Príncipe A, Dib E, Freymuller E, Moraes N, Farah ME: Effects of subretinal injection of patent blue and trypan blue in rabbits. Curr Eye Res 2007;32:309–317.

Eduardo B. Rodrigues, MD
Rua Presidente Coutinho 579, conj 501
Florianópolis, SC 88015–300 (Brazil)
Tel./Fax +55 48 3222 3380, E-Mail edubrodriguess@yahoo.com.br

Meyer CH (ed): Vital Dyes in Vitreoretinal Surgery.
Dev Ophthalmol. Basel, Karger, 2008, vol 42, pp 101–114

Trityl Dyes Patent Blue V and Brilliant Blue G – Clinical Relevance and in vitro Analysis of the Function of the Outer Blood-Retinal Barrier

Stefan Mennel[a] · Carsten H. Meyer[b] · Jörg C. Schmidt[a] · Stefanie Kaempf[c] · Gabriele Thumann[c,d]

[a]Department of Ophthalmology, Philipps-University Marburg, Marburg, [b]Department of Ophthalmology, University Bonn, Bonn, [c]IZKF 'Biomat', and [d]Department of Ophthalmology, Rheinisch-Westfälische Technische Hochschule Aachen, Aachen, Germany

Abstract

The use of vital dyes during vitrectomy allows easier removal of less recognizable structures like epiretinal membranes or the internal limiting membrane (ILM). In recent years, numerous studies have investigated the use of indocyanine green (ICG), trypan blue (Membrane Blue™), triamcinolone, autologous blood and presently trityl dyes such as patent blue V (PBV, Blueron™), crystal violet and brilliant blue G (BBG, Brilliant Peel™) in chromovitrectomy. Reports on potential risks of these dyes, especially ICG, such as reduced visual acuity, possible visual field defects or alterations of the retinal pigment epithelium (RPE) limited their application. A systematic review of the literature up to July 2007 was performed using Medline (http://www.ncbi.nlm.nih.gov/PubMed/) where we specifically searched for relevant information regarding the laboratory as well as clinical use of PB and BBG. To evaluate the effect of PB and BBG on the RPE, PB and BBG have been added to an in vitro model of the outer blood-retinal barrier to assess dye-associated barrier properties. Two concentrations of PB (2.4 and 1.2 mg/ml) and BBG (0.25 and 2.4 mg/ml) were investigated. To simulate in vivo conditions of a fluid-filled eye and an air-filled eye the dyes were added either to the culture medium or directly to the RPE cells where they remained for 2.5 min. To determine barrier properties, transepithelial resistance (TER) was measured at 3 days of follow-up. Ultrastructural integrity of RPE cells was evaluated by transmission electron microscopy. Following application of PB, barrier properties in the fluid- as well as in the air-filled eye showed only mild, transient and no significant decrease in TER. BBG did not cause a breakdown of the outer blood-retinal barrier at the concentration of 0.25 mg/ml in the model of the fluid-filled eye. The concentration of 2.4 mg/ml in the model of the fluid-filled eye as well as both concentrations in the model of the air-filled eye showed a minor decrease after 1.5 h, which was no longer observed after 24 h. Transmission electron microscopy did not show any dye-associated ultrastructural alterations to the RPE cells. In clinical use, PB showed only mild staining of epiretinal membranes and moderate staining of the ILM. Although BBG did not stain epiretinal membranes, it represents an appropriate candidate for the future, as BBG has a high affinity for the ILM. The use of trityl dyes in the posterior eye segment seems to be safe concerning damage to the RPE and its barrier function, especially when the dye is applied to the fluid-filled eye.

The use of vital dyes during vitrectomy allows visualization and easier removal of less recognizable, semitransparent structures like epiretinal membranes or the internal limiting membrane (ILM) [1]. Numerous studies have investigated the use of indocyanine green (ICG), trypan blue (TB, Membrane Blue™), triamcinolone, autologous blood and presently trityl dyes such as patent blue V (PBV, Blueron™), crystal violet and brilliant blue G (BBG, Brilliant Peel™) in chromovitrectomy [2–8]. As reported, these dyes, especially ICG, could cause reduced visual acuity, possible visual field defects or alterations of the retinal pigment epithelium (RPE) [9–11].

Theoretically, dyes could provoke toxicity to the RPE in full-thickness macular holes or due to diffusion of the dye through the neuroretina.

The RPE consists of a monolayer of polarized hexagonal cells densely adherent to one another through a system of tight cellular junctions that surround the apical part of the cells. Because they obstruct the paracellular route, they are also called zonulae occludentes. Together with the endothelium of the choriocapillaris and Bruch's membrane they build the outer blood-retinal barrier, which is similar structurally and functionally to the blood-brain barrier [12]. The RPE plays an essential role in maintaining viability and functionality of the neural retina and, among other functions, prevents the neurosensory retina from accumulating extracellular fluid in the subretinal space and degrades and recycles receptor outer segments and thus prevents deposition of debris in the subretinal space [13]. Damage to the RPE would result in disruption of the blood-retinal barrier and impairment of neural retina function.

RPE changes have been observed after the intraoperative use of ICG [14, 15]. As a consequence, several studies evaluated the functional and anatomical results after ICG-assisted ILM peeling demonstrating controversial results [9, 16–20]. Animal models were used exhibiting a dose-dependent mechanism of ICG toxicity to the RPE [21–23]. Additionally, an in vitro analysis showed a dose-dependent cytotoxic influence of ICG on RPE cell activity and cell morphology [24, 25].

Alternative dyes are designed with adequate properties to safely stain the ILM and/or epiretinal membranes in vivo. PBV (Blueron; Fluoron, Neu-Ulm, Germany and Geuder, Heidelberg, Germany) and BBG (Brilliant Peel; Fluoron and Geuder) are two new synthetic dyes of the trityl dye group that are currently evaluated in laboratory tests as well as in clinical trials.

PBV, also called food blue 5 or sulfan blue, is a disulfonated diaminotriphenylmethane ($C_{27}H_{31}N_2O_7S_2Na$) and has served for decades as a frequently used vital dye in textiles, cosmetics, agriculture and numerous medical products (E131). Moreover, it has been applied for a long time as a biological stain to study fluid movement in the kidney and more recently to perform lymphangiography. In oncology, PBV is also frequently used as a sensitive marker to facilitate the complete excision of affected lymph nodes [26, 27]. If used intraocularly, PBV is applied at a concentration of 2.4 mg/ml.

BBG ($C_{47}N_{48}N_3O_7S_2Na$, Coomassie™ G250, acid blue 90) is also called food blue 2 (E133). It is used as a food color, in soaps, shampoos and cosmetics. BBG may also be applied as a marker in cardiovascular and neurological diseases. It is soluble in water with a maximum absorption at about 630 nm [27, 28]. In ophthalmology, BBG is applied at a concentration of 0.25 mg/ml.

Several parameters are sensitive to evaluate cytotoxicity: cell viability, cell activity, cell count, light and electron microscopy to show morphologic alterations, as well as transepithelial resistance (TER) that measures integrity of the outer blood retinal-barrier function [29, 30]. Following a review of the literature concerning in vitro as well as in vivo use of PB and BBG, we studied the effects of these two dyes in an in vitro cell model of fluid- and air-filled eyes [31, 32]. Additionally, transmission electron microscopy was used to describe ultrastructural findings.

Materials and Methods

A systematic review of the literature up to July 2007 was performed using Medline (http://www.ncbi.nlm.nih.gov/PubMed/) where we specifically searched for relevant information regarding laboratory investigations, animal trials as well as clinical use of PB and BBG.

All experiments were performed with ARPE-19 (LGC Promochem GmbH, Wesel, Germany), a human diploid RPE cell line, which is in many aspects similar to the RPE in vivo [33]. Passage 17 was used for our experiments. Before seeding, the cells were washed and then incubated with trypsin/EDTA (0.05%/0.02%; PAA Laboratories GmbH, Pasching, Germany) for 5 min at 37°C; after trypsin was inactivated by fetal bovine serum gold, the cells were collected by centrifugation at 1,000 U/min for 10 min. Cells were cultured in Dulbecco's modified Eagle's medium/Ham's F-12 (1:1; Biochrom AG, Berlin, Germany) supplemented with antibiotics (streptomycin and penicillin; Lonza, Verviers, Belgium) and 10% fetal bovine serum gold at 37°C in a humidified atmosphere of 5% CO_2/95% air. Medium was changed every 72 h.

To measure TER, ARPE-19 cells were seeded at a density of 45,000 cells/cm^2 on 0.4-μm pore-sized semipermeable polycarbonate membranes with a 0.6-cm^2 effective surface area (Millicell®-PCF, Millipore Corporation, Bedford, Mass., USA) cultured in the above-described culture medium. Cell viability and confluent growth were monitored in a control group, cultured on a plastic petri dish. At confluence, the serum concentration of the culture medium was reduced to 1% [34]. In a previous study, we evaluated the influence of human endothelial cells on the outer blood-retinal barrier in an in vitro model. The results have shown that endothelial cells of the choroid could not be used in this in vitro model of the outer blood-retinal barrier, because they are not able to establish a TER [32].

In a previous experiment, we determined TER by using electrode measurement and confluent growth and found a TER of 25–40 Ω cm^2 3 weeks after seeding on the permeable membranes. Obtaining two stable values on 2 subsequent days after this time period allowed us to assume the formation of a tightly coupled cell monolayer. The effects of BBG, PB as well as ICG were evaluated and compared with trypsin as a control.

Because TER measurements were carried out over a 3-day period and required identical positioning of the electrodes, we optimized reproducibility and stability by using an epithelial voltohmmeter and the Endohm-12 chamber (World Precision Instruments, Sarasota, Fla., USA), a device with fixed electrodes [32]. The bottom of this chamber as well as the cap at the top of the chamber contain a pair of concentric electrodes that incorporate a voltage-sensing Ag/AgCl pellet in the center and an annular current electrode. The Millipore culture cup with a confluent monolayer of ARPE-19 cells was placed into the Endohm-12 chamber to determine TER.

To measure the resistance of the naked Millicell-PCF and the culture medium, 2 ml of culture medium were placed in the Endohm-12 chamber (basal medium). Constant medium volume in all experiments was achieved by the use of 300 µl of Dulbecco's modified Eagle's medium as an apical medium for TER measurements. To quantify TER of the RPE monolayer, the resistance values of the medium and the naked filter were subtracted, and the result multiplied by the area of the inserts.

Two different models representing an air-filled and a fluid-filled eye were tested by adding the dye to the culture medium (50 µl of the apical medium were replaced by 50 µl of the dye) or by directly applying it on the cell monolayer after removal of the apical medium. In these two models, PB (2.4 and 1.2 mg/ml) and BBG (0.25 and 2.4 mg/ml) were applied for 2.5 min and the influence on the barrier function was determined by TER measured prior to as well as 1.5 h, 3 h, 1 day, 3 days and 7 days after dye exposure. As a control group, TER was measured without dye application but with fluid (culture medium) exchange to simulate the effect of mechanic stress due to the maneuvers. Additionally, TER was measured after applying ICG (5 mg/ml) for 2.5 min as well as trypsin/EDTA (0.05%/0.02%) for 12 min at 37°C. Each experiment was done in triplicate.

Transmission electron microscopy was performed after direct exposure of RPE cells to PB and BBG for 2.5 min. Specimens of monolayers were obtained by cutting out the membranes from the Millicell-PCF. The specimens were fixated in 3% glutaraldehyde in 0.1 M sodium cacodylate buffer (pH 7.4), postfixated in Dalton's fixative, dehydrated through a graded ethanol series and embedded in Epon. Semithin sections were stained with methylene blue. Ultrathin sections were contrasted with 1.5% uranyl acetate and analyzed using an electron microscope.

Results

The systematic review of the literature regarding laboratory investigations, animal trials as well as clinical use of PB and BBG showed only 5 papers for PB and 5 papers for BBG. These articles are summarized in table 1 (BBG) and table 2 (PB).

Effectivity and reproducibility of the in vitro model of the outer blood-retinal barrier using the Endohm-12 device have been shown in a previous publication [32].

First, in a control group, culture medium was replaced as in the experiments but without dyes to demonstrate the influence of this manipulation on TER. The initial mean TER of 37.2 Ω cm^2 (range: 36.6–38.4) changed to 36 Ω cm^2 (mean; range: 34.8–37.2) after 1.5 h, 38 Ω cm^2 (mean; range: 36–40.2) after 3 h, 39.4 Ω cm^2 (mean; range: 38.4–40.2) after 24 h and 37 Ω cm^2 (mean; range: 34.8–38.4) after 3 days (fig. 1).

Second, trypsin/EDTA (0.05%/0.02%) was applied for 12 min at 37°C and TER was followed up for 3 days. The initial TER of 35.6 Ω cm^2 (mean; range: 33–39.6) changed to 10.8 Ω cm^2 (mean; range: 9.6–12.6) after 12 min, 15.6 Ω cm^2 (mean; range: 15–16.8) after 1.5 h, 17 Ω cm^2 (mean; range: 16.2–18.6) after 3 h, 20.6 Ω cm^2 (mean; range: 18.6–24) after 24 h and 24.8 Ω cm^2 (mean; range: 22.2–28.2) after 3 days (fig. 1).

Third, an additional control was performed by the application of ICG (5 mg/ml) for 2.5 min. The initial TER of 36.6 Ω cm^2 (mean; range: 34.8–37.8) changed to 31.6 Ω cm^2 (mean; range: 30.6–32.4) after 1.5 h, 32.8 Ω cm^2 (mean; range: 30.6–36) after 3 h, 37.2 Ω cm^2 (mean; range: 34.8–39) after 24 h and 39.2 Ω cm^2 (mean; range: 37.8–40.2) after 3 days (fig. 1).

Table 1. Review of the literature: safety studies of BBG on the RPE and clinical experience

Authors	Concentration	Study design	Results, effect on human RPE cells
Ueno et al. [41]	0.25 mg/ml	subretinal injection in a rat model, evaluation over 2 months and 2 weeks	in comparison to ICG and TB, there was no cytotoxic effect of BBG on the retina and RPE
Enaida et al. [40]	10, 5, 1, and 0.01 mg/ml	rat model, BBG intravitreal injection for 2 weeks and 2 months, BBG solution	high doses of BBG (1.0 and 10 mg/ml) induced vacuolization in the inner retinal cells, but apoptosis was not detected
Hisatomi et al. [39]	10, 1.0, 0.5, 0.25, 0.1, and 0.01 mg/ml	rat eyes for 2 months	no apparent toxic effect was observed using biomicroscopy during 2 months
Enaida et al. [42]	0.25 mg/ml	human: BBG solution into the vitreous cavity and immediate washout (20 eyes)	BBG selectively stains the ILM, not ERM
Cervera et al. [4]	0.5 mg/ml	human: BBG solution into the vitreous cavity and immediate washout (6 eyes)	BBG stains the ILM with high affinity

ERM = Epiretinal membrane.

PB was applied at two concentrations in the model of the fluid- and air-filled eye. When PB was added at a concentration of 1.2 mg/ml in the model of the air-filled eye, the initial TER of 36.8 $\Omega\,cm^2$ (mean; range: 36.6–37.2) changed to 31.2 $\Omega\,cm^2$ (mean; range: 30.6–31.8) after 1.5 h, 32 $\Omega\,cm^2$ (mean; range: 31.2–33.6) after 3 h, 38.6 $\Omega\,cm^2$ (mean; range: 38.4–39) after 24 h and 37.2 $\Omega\,cm^2$ (mean; range: 35.4–38.4) after 3 days. When the concentration of 1.2 mg/ml was used in the model of the fluid-filled eye, the initial TER of 38.6 $\Omega\,cm^2$ (mean; range: 38.4–39) changed to 33.4 $\Omega\,cm^2$ (mean; range: 32.4–34.2) after 1.5 h, 33.4 $\Omega\,cm^2$ (mean; range: 31.8–34.2) after 3 h, 39.4 $\Omega\,cm^2$ (mean; range: 38.4–40.2) after 24 h and 39 $\Omega\,cm^2$ (mean; range: 37.2–41.4) after 3 days (fig. 2).

When PB was added at a concentration of 2.4 mg/ml in the model of the air-filled eye, the initial TER of 36.8 $\Omega\,cm^2$ (mean; range: 36–38.4) changed to 33.8 $\Omega\,cm^2$ (mean; range: 33–34.8) after 1.5 h, 34 $\Omega\,cm^2$ (mean; range: 33.6–34.2) after 3 h, 38 $\Omega\,cm^2$ (mean; range: 37.2–38.4) after 24 h and 37 $\Omega\,cm^2$ (mean; range: 36.6–37.2) after 3 days. When the concentration of 2.4 mg/ml was added in the model of the fluid-filled eye, the initial TER of 36.2 $\Omega\,cm^2$ (mean; range: 35.4–37.2) changed to 35.8 $\Omega\,cm^2$ (mean; range: 35.4–36) after 1.5 h, 35.8 $\Omega\,cm^2$ (mean; range: 34.2–39) after 3 h, 34.6 $\Omega\,cm^2$ (mean; range: 34.2–34.8) after 24 h and 34.9 $\Omega\,cm^2$ (mean; range: 34–35.4) after 3 days (fig. 2).

Table 2. Review of the literature: safety studies of PB on the RPE and clinical experience

Authors	Concentration	Study design	Results, effect on human RPE cells
Maia et al. [38]	2.4 mg/ml	subretinal injection in a rabbit model; 2.4 mg/ml PB; 6, 12 and 24 h and 14 days	subretinal injection of PB caused POS and PIS abnormalities 12 and 24 h after surgery as well as ONL damage 14 days after surgery
Luke et al. [36]	0.48%	bovine retinal ERG model; PB application time: varied between 10 s and 2 min (10, 15, 30, 60, 120 s)	loss of the b-wave was only seen for an exposure period of 120 s; the effects of PB on the ERG was completely reversible
Luke et al. [37]	0.48%	human retinal ERG model, PB application time: 15 s to 4 min	no effects on the human ERG were seen after 15 and 30 s of dye application; reversible reductions of the b-wave amplitude were found for an exposure period of 60 and 120 s; after 4 min of PB application, a persistent b-wave amplitude reduction by 40% was found
Mennel et al. [32]	2.4 and 0.24 mg/ml	3 min to culture medium and directly to the RPE cells, applied for 3 min to the outer blood-retinal barrier in an in vitro model	PB had no influence on the outer blood-retinal barrier function and growth characteristics of RPE cells
Mennel et al. [6]	2.4 mg/ml	human: PB solution into the vitreous cavity and immediate washout	only mild staining of ERM, moderate staining of the ILM with fast vanishing of the dye

POS = Photoreceptor outer segment; PIS = photoreceptor inner segment; ONL = outer nuclear layer; ERM = epiretinal membrane.

BBG was applied at two concentrations in the model of the fluid- and air-filled eye. When BBG was added at a concentration of 0.25 mg/ml in the model of the air-filled eye, the initial TER of 38.6 $\Omega\,cm^2$ (mean; range: 37.2–39.6) changed to 32.4 $\Omega\,cm^2$ (mean; range: 30.6–34.2) after 1.5 h, 33.2 $\Omega\,cm^2$ (mean; range: 30.6–34.8) after 3 h, 38.4 $\Omega\,cm^2$ (mean; range: 34.8–40.2) after 24 h and 37.2 $\Omega\,cm^2$ (mean) after 3 days. When the concentration of 0.25 mg/ml was added in the model of the fluid-filled eye, the initial TER of 35.8 $\Omega\,cm^2$ (mean; range: 34.8–37.2) changed to 33.4 $\Omega\,cm^2$ (mean; range: 32.4–34.8) after 1.5 h, 34 $\Omega\,cm^2$ (mean; range: 33.6–34.2) after 3 h, 35.8 $\Omega\,cm^2$ (mean; range: 35.4–36) after 24 h and 37.6 $\Omega\,cm^2$ (mean; range: 36–39) after 3 days (fig. 3).

When BBG was added at a concentration of 2.4 mg/ml in the model of the air-filled eye, the initial TER of 38.0 $\Omega\,cm^2$ (mean; range: 35.4–39.6) changed to 31.6 $\Omega\,cm^2$ (mean; range: 29.4–33) after 1.5 h, 32.4 $\Omega\,cm^2$ (mean; range: 31.2–33.6)

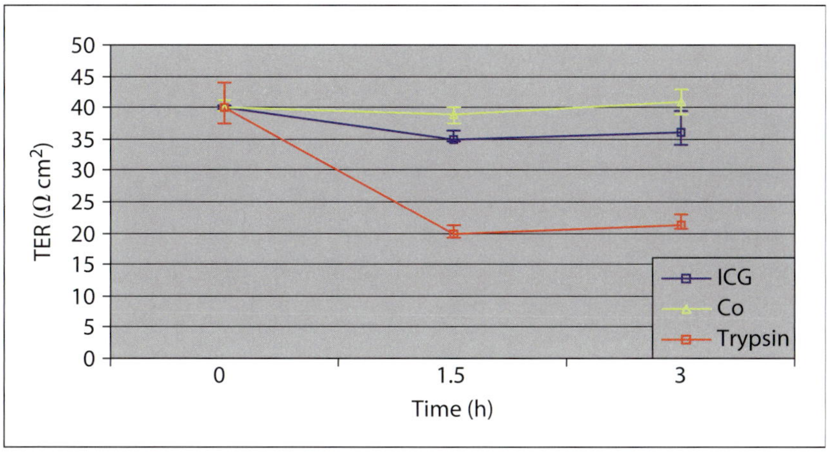

Fig. 1. TER within 3 h. Three control groups were used: (1) without dye (Co), (2) with 5 mg/ml ICG and (3) with trypsin/EDTA (0.05%/0.02%). The mean TER at the beginning of the experiments was standardized to 40 Ω cm^2 to compare equal values.

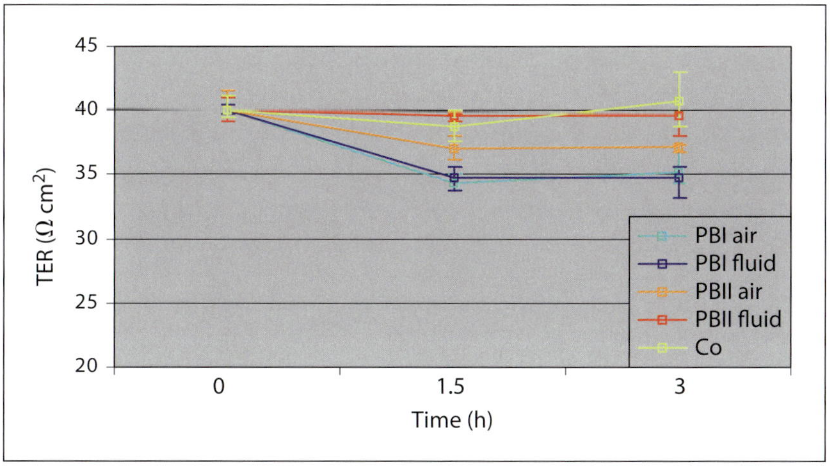

Fig. 2. TER within 3 h. PB was used at a concentration of 1.2 mg/ml (PBI) and 2.4 mg/ml (PBII) in the model of the fluid- and air-filled eye. The scale of the y-axis has been limited from 20 to 45 Ω cm^2. The mean TER at the beginning of the experiments was standardized to 40 Ω cm^2 to compare equal values.

after 3 h, 35.2 Ω cm^2 (mean; range: 32.4–36.6) after 24 h and 34.4 Ω cm^2 (mean; range: 31.2–36) after 3 days. When the concentration of 2.4 mg/ml was added in the model of the fluid-filled eye, the initial TER of 37.4 Ω cm^2 (mean; range: 35.4–38.4) changed to 32.4 Ω cm^2 (mean; range: 30.6–33.6) after 1.5 h, 36.6 Ω cm^2 (mean; range: 31.2–38.4) after 3 h, 36.8 Ω cm^2 (mean; range: 36.6–37.2) after 24 h and 34.2 Ω cm^2 (mean; range: 33–34.8) after 3 days (fig. 3).

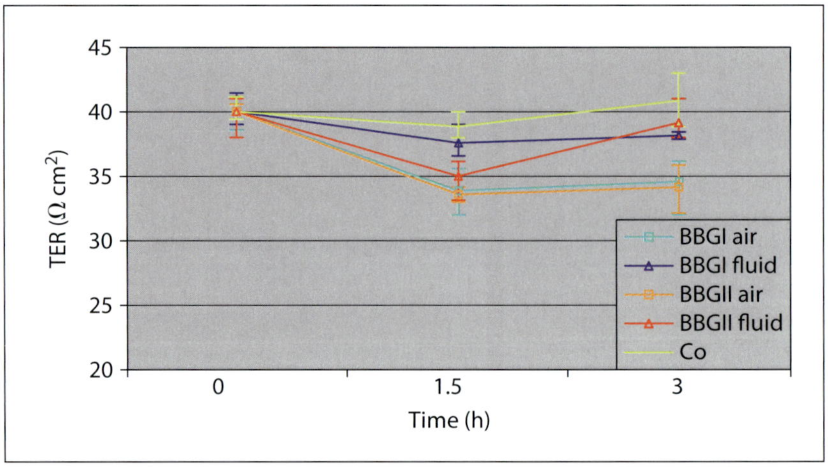

Fig. 3. TER within 3 h. BBG was used at a concentration of 0.25 mg/ml (BBGI) and 2.4 mg/ml (BBGII) in the model of the fluid- and air-filled eye. The scale of the y-axis has been limited from 20 to 45 Ω cm^2. The mean TER at the beginning of the experiments was standardized to 40 Ω cm^2 to compare equal values.

Transmission electron microscopy revealed normal cell morphology as well as normal intercellular adhesion with desmosomes and tight junctions. No dye-related ultrastructural alterations were visible with both concentrations of PB and BBG following the direct application of the dye to the RPE cells. The mitochondria, i.e. cell organelles sensitive to any cell damage, did not show swelling or other structural changes, nor did the intracellular matrix, nucleus or cell membrane (fig. 4a–d).

Discussion

Our in vitro analysis showed that in the control groups trypsin/EDTA (0.05%/0.02%), applied for 10 min, caused an immediate breakdown of the blood-retinal barrier. The application of ICG (5 mg/ml) induced a moderate and transient decrease in TER within 24 h. Similar results for ICG had already been demonstrated in a previous publication [32]. An additional control group without the use of dyes but with the exchange of fluid to simulate the effect of mechanic stress due to the maneuvers showed stable TER at 3 days of follow-up (fig. 1).

Patent Blue

After the application of PB, barrier properties showed only a mild and no significant decrease in TER. Interestingly, the mean decrease in TER was greater (5.2 Ω cm^2,

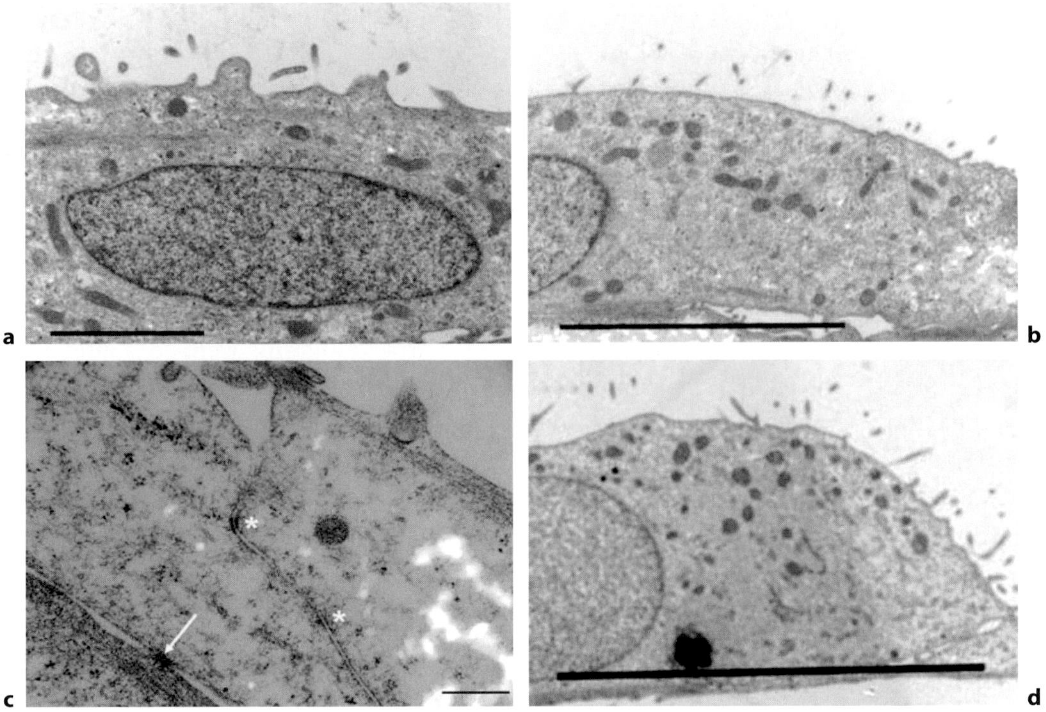

Fig. 4. a–d Transmission electron microscopy. **a** After application of PB (1.2 mg/ml), no morphological alterations of the RPE cells could be observed and the typical microvilli are visible (top of the image, magnification bar = 2 μm). **b** After application of BBG (0.25 mg/ml), the cell morphology appears normal and microvilli are visible (top of the image, magnification bar = 5 μm). **c** After exposure to BBG (2.4 mg/ml), the cell adhesions with desmosomes (arrow) and tight junctions (asterisks) do not present any dye-related ultrastructural signs of outer blood-retinal barrier breakdown (magnification bar = 500 nm). **d** Normal cell morphology of the RPE cell with microvilli at the apical cell following exposure to BBG (2.4 mg/ml; magnification bar = 10 μm).

fluid-filled eye) in the group with the lower concentration (1.2 mg/ml) compared to the higher concentration (2.4 mg/ml). At this concentration, the mean decrease was only 0.4 $\Omega\,cm^2$ in the fluid-filled eye. Additionally, there was no significant difference between the air- and fluid-filled eye experiments. In summary, PB at both concentrations did not significantly influence TER in the fluid- as well as in the air-filled eye (fig. 2). Transmission electron microscopy revealed no structural changes of the cells, cell compartments and intercellular structures.

Safety studies for the intraocular use of PB have been reported by Hiebl et al. [35], demonstrating that cytotoxic effects occur only at concentrations 10–20 times higher than the recommended PB concentration to visualize intraocular structures such as the anterior capsule during cataract surgery. Animal experiments by Luke et al. [36] investigated the effect of PB 0.48% and compared this to ICG 0.05% and TB 0.15%

on bovine retina by electroretinography (ERG). PB 0.48% and ICG 0.05% showed completely reversible effects for an exposure duration of up to 120 s. However, TB induced a reversible loss of the b-wave for an exposure of 10 s or less. A slightly prolonged exposure time of 15 s caused a significant b-wave reduction, which was only partially reversible during the recovery time. The authors concluded that the intraocular application of PB 0.48% and ICG 0.05% 'seems to be safe' with a short incubation and limited duration in the eye [36]. For further studies, Luke et al. [37] isolated human retina prepared and perfused with a standard solution, and ERG was performed repeatedly. The solution was substituted by PB for a duration that varied between 15 s and 4 min. No effects on human electroretinograms were seen after 15 and 30 s of dye application. Reversible reductions of the b-wave amplitude were found for an exposure period of 60 and 120 s. After 4 min of PB application, a persistent b-wave amplitude reduction by 40% was found. The authors concluded that PB affects human retinal function when applied for at least 1 min. However, no irreversible effects on human electroretinograms were seen even after 2 min of retinal exposure to PB. Maia et al. [38] investigated the histological and clinical effects of subretinal injection of 2.4 mg/ml PB and TB in rabbits. Histological evaluation disclosed only minimal abnormalities on the photoreceptor outer segment after subretinal injection of balanced salt solution during all follow-ups. Subretinal injection of PB caused photoreceptor outer segment and photoreceptor inner segment abnormalities 12 and 24 h after surgery as well as outer nuclear layer damage 14 days after surgery. Subretinal injection of TB induced more significant clinical and histological damage to the neurosensory retina/RPE than did PB or balanced salt solution [38].

Brilliant Blue G

Our in vitro analysis of BBG did not show a breakdown of the outer blood-retinal barrier properties at the concentration of 0.25 mg/ml in the model of the fluid-filled eye. At the concentration of 2.4 mg/ml in the model of the fluid-filled eye, there was only a minor decrease after 1.5 h, which was not detectable 3 h after exposure. In the model of the air-filled eye, both concentrations (0.25 and 2.4 mg/ml) showed a moderate decrease in TER after 1.5 and 3 h. The difference between the mean TER of the control group and the mean TER of the BBG group at the concentration of 0.25 mg/ml was 5.0 $\Omega\,cm^2$ after 1.5 h and 6.2 $\Omega\,cm^2$ after 3 h, and at the concentration of 2.4 mg/ml the difference was 5.2 $\Omega\,cm^2$ after 1.5 h and 6.6 $\Omega\,cm^2$ after 3 h (fig. 3). After 24 h, there was no difference between the control group and the BBG group at both concentrations. Transmission electron microscopy revealed no structural changes of the cells, cell compartments and intercellular structures. The limitations of our experiments and in general are that the results of in vitro analyses do not exactly represent in vivo conditions in human beings. Although each experiment was done in triplicate, the range of the results did not demonstrate a toxic effect of BBG in the model of the air-filled eye, as there was only a moderate and transient decrease in the mean TER. For clinical use, the lower concentration of 0.25 mg/ml is available. Additionally, most surgeons today use vital dyes to visualize preretinal and retinal structures in the fluid-filled eye. In the model of the fluid-filled eye, no significant alteration in the control group could be found.

Safety studies for the intraocular use of BBG have been reported by Hisatomi et al. [39] evaluating the effectiveness and biocompatibility of BBG for capsular visualization. In rat eyes, no damage including apoptotic cell death or degeneration of corneal endothelial cells has been observed in the long-term observation period of 2 months. Enaida et al. [40] investigated the effect of intravitreal BBG on the morphology and function of the retina and its possible use for staining and peeling of the ILM. In rat eyes (n = 78), BBG solution was injected into the vitreous cavity. The eyes were enucleated at 2 weeks and 2 months. In the rat eyes, no pathologic changes were observed with light microscopy. Electron microscopy revealed that high doses of BBG induced vacuolization in the inner retinal cells, but apoptosis was not detected. There was no reduction in the amplitude of the ERG waves, indicating that BBG has a low potential for toxicity. Using a rat model, Ueno et al. [41] injected BBG (0.25 mg/ml) subretinally and its effect was evaluated over 2 months and 2 weeks. The results were compared with those for ICG (5 mg/ml) and TB (1 mg/ml). Whereas ICG and TB caused retinal degeneration and RPE cell atrophy 2 weeks after subretinal injection, BBG showed no detectable toxic effects after 2 months and 2 weeks.

In clinical use, PB shows only mild staining of epiretinal membranes and moderate staining of the ILM [6]. The 'dusty' appearance and the fast vanishing of the dye indicate only a mild adhesion to the retinal surface (fig. 5). Enaida et al. [42] demonstrated a sufficiently improved visualization of the ILM by BBG enabling peeling and surgery to be performed successfully (fig. 6). Staining of the epiretinal membranes could not be confirmed for BBG at a concentration 0.25 mg/ml. In this interventional, noncomparative, prospective, clinical case series of 20 eyes from 20 consecutive patients with macular holes or epiretinal membranes, no adverse effects were observed postoperatively during the observation period (mean follow-up ± SD, 7.3 ± 1.0 months). Cervera et al. [4] used BBG to enhance visualization of the ILM during vitrectomy in humans and demonstrated that BBG was a very helpful dye to enhance visualization of the ILM.

In summary, the use of trityl dyes in the posterior eye segment seems to be safe concerning damage to the RPE and its barrier function, especially when the dye is used in the fluid-filled eye. Whereas the dye accumulates in the air-filled eye, the concentrations are immediately reduced by dilution of the dye in the fluid-filled eye. Additionally, a short time of dye application reduces possible toxic side effects. In clinical practice, BBG stains the ILM with high affinity and therefore arises as the first real alternative option to ICG and infracyanine green in chromovitrectomy, although limited toxicity data on BBG application still warrant further investigations.

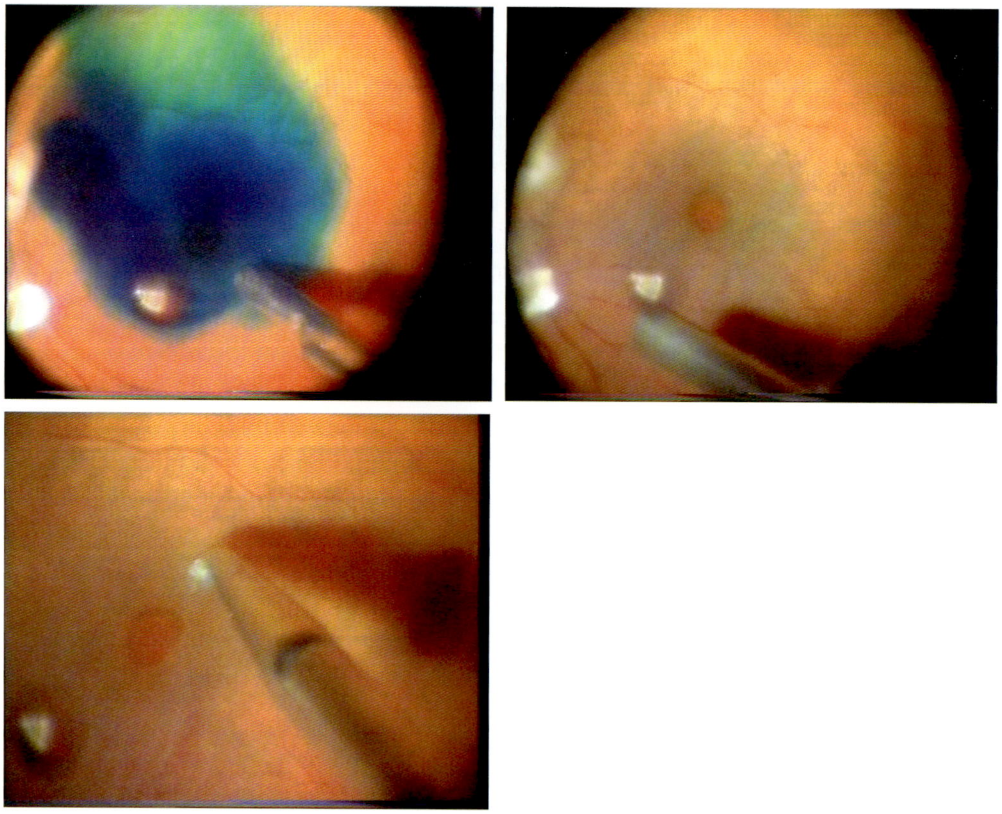

Fig. 5. a–c PB staining of the ILM in a case of macular hole. Following immediate aspiration of the dye, ILM peeling was performed. There is only moderate PB staining of the ILM.

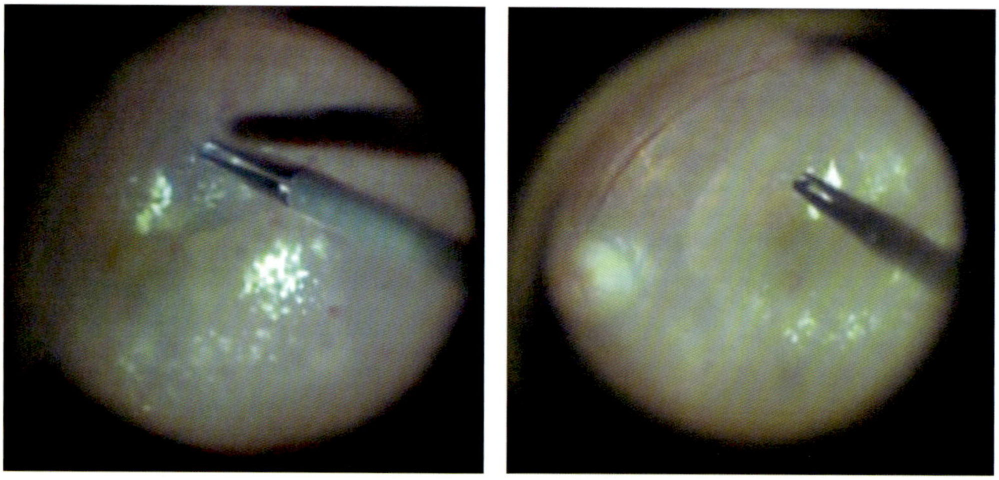

Fig. 6. a, **b** ILM peeling after staining with BBG in a case of diabetic macular edema. Courtesy of Hiroshi Enaida, MD.

Acknowledgments

This work has been supported by the Fehr Foundation, Marburg, Germany, and by a grant from the Interdisciplinary Center for Clinical Research 'Biomat.' within the Faculty of Medicine at the Rheinisch-Westfälische Technische Hochschule Aachen, Germany. The authors acknowledge Prof. Dr. P. Walter (Chair of the Department of Ophthalmology, University of Aachen) for the use of laboratory facilities, Christiane Maltusch (Laboratory for Experimental Ophthalmology, University of Aachen) for her assistance in the culture of RPE cells and in vitro analysis, and Hiroshi Enaida, MD, and Tatsuro Ishibashi, MD, for the image demonstrating the high affinity of BBG for the ILM.

References

1 Rodrigues EB, Meyer CH, Kroll P: Chromovitrectomy: a new field in vitreoretinal surgery. Graefes Arch Clin Exp Ophthalmol 2005;243:291–293.

2 Eshita T, Inoue M, Kazuto Y, Shinoda K, Ishida S: Indocyanine green can distinguish posterior vitreous cortex from internal limiting membrane during vitrectomy with removal of epiretinal membrane. Retina 2002;22:104–106.

3 Gandorfer A, Messmer EM, Ulbig MW, Kampik A: Indocyanine green selectively stains the internal limiting membrane. Am J Ophthalmol 2001;131:387–388.

4 Cervera E, Diaz-Llopis M, Salom D, Udaondo P, Amselem L: Internal limiting membrane staining using intravitreal brilliant blue G: good help for vitreo-retinal surgeon in training. Arch Soc Esp Oftalmol 2007;82: 71–72.

5 Schmidt JC, Meyer CH, Rodrigues EB, Hörle S, Kroll P: Staining of internal limiting membrane in vitreomacular surgery: a simplified technique. Retina 2003;23:263–264.

6 Mennel S, Meyer CH, Tietjen A, Rodrigues EB, Schmidt JC: Patent blue: a novel vital dye in vitreoretinal surgery. Ophthalmologica 2006;220:190–193.

7 Enaida H, Hisatomi T, Goto Y, Hata Y, Ueno A, Miura M, Kubota T, Ishibashi T: Preclinical investigation of internal limiting membrane staining and peeling using intravitreal brilliant blue G. Retina 2006;26:623–630.

8 Matsumoto H, Yamanaka I, Hisatomi T, Enaida H, Ueno A, Hata Y, Sakamoto T, Ogino N, Ishibashi T: Triamcinolone acetonide-assisted pars plana vitrectomy improves residual posterior vitreous hyaloid removal: ultrastructural analysis of the inner limiting membrane. Retina 2007;27:174–179.

9 Kanda S, Uemura A, Yamashita T, Kita H, Yamakiri K, Sakamoto T: Visual field defects after intravitreous administration of indocyanine green in macular hole surgery. Arch Ophthalmol 2004;122:1447–1451.

10 Kusaka S, Oshita T, Ohji M, Tano Y: Reduction of the toxic effect of indocyanine green on retinal pigment epithelium during macular hole surgery. Retina 2003;23:733–734.

11 Maia M, Haller JA, Pieramici DJ, Margalit E, de Juan E Jr, Farah ME, Lakhanpal RR, Eong KG, Guven D, Humayun MS: Retinal pigment epithelial abnormalities after internal limiting membrane peeling guided by indocyanine green staining. Retina 2004; 24:157–160.

12 Raviola G: The structural basis of the blood-ocular barriers. Exp Eye Res 1977;25(suppl):27–63.

13 Marmor MF: Control of subretinal fluid: experimental and clinical studies. Eye 1990;4:340–344.

14 Engelbrecht NE, Freeman J, Sternberg P Jr, Aaberg TM Sr, Aaberg TM Jr, Martin DF, Sippy BD: Retinal pigment epithelial changes after macular hole surgery with indocyanine green-assisted internal limiting membrane peeling. Am J Ophthalmol 2002; 133:89–94.

15 Sakamoto T, Itaya K, Noda Y, Ishibashi T: Retinal pigment epithelial changes after indocyanine green-assisted vitrectomy. Retina 2002;22:794–796.

16 Ando F, Sasano K, Ohba N, Hirose H, Yasui O: Anatomic and visual outcomes after indocyanine green-assisted peeling of the retinal internal limiting membrane in idiopathic macular hole surgery. Am J Ophthalmol 2004;137:744–746.

17 Gandorfer A, Haritoglou C, Gass CA, Ulbig MW, Kampik A: Indocyanine green-assisted peeling of the internal limiting membrane may cause retinal damage. Am J Ophthalmol 2001;132:431–433.

18 Gass CA, Haritoglou C, Schaumberger M, Kampik A: Functional outcome of macular hole surgery with and without indocyanine green-assisted peeling of the internal limiting membrane. Graefes Arch Clin Exp Ophthalmol 2003;241:716–720.

19 Grisanti S, Szurman P, Gelisken F, Aisenbrey S, Oficjalska-Mlynczak J, Bartz-Schmidt KU: Histological findings in experimental macular surgery with indocyanine green. Invest Ophthalmol Vis Sci 2004;45:282–286.

20 Haritoglou C, Gandorfer A, Gass CA, Schaumberger M, Ulbig MW, Kampik A: Indocyanine green-assisted peeling of the internal limiting membrane in macular hole surgery affects visual outcome: a clinicopathologic correlation. Am J Ophthalmol 2002; 134:836–841.
21 Czajka MP, McCuen BW 2nd, Cummings TJ, Nguyen H, Stinnett S, Wong F: Effects of indocyanine green on the retina and retinal pigment epithelium in a porcine model of retinal hole. Retina 2004;24: 275–282.
22 Ho JD, Tsai RJ, Chen SN, Chen HC: Cytotoxicity of indocyanine green on retinal pigment epithelium. Arch Ophthalmol 2003;121:1423–1429.
23 Kawaji T, Hirata A, Inomata Y, Koga T, Tanihara H: Morphological damage in rabbit retina caused by subretinal injection of indocyanine green. Graefes Arch Clin Exp Ophthalmol 2004;242:158–164.
24 Gale JS, Proulx AA, Gonder JR, Mao AJ, Hutnik CM: Comparison of the in vitro toxicity of indocyanine green to that of trypan blue in human retinal pigment epithelium cell cultures. Am J Ophthalmol 2004;138:64–69.
25 Rezai KA, Farrokh-Siar L, Ernest JT, van Seventer GA: Indocyanine green induces apoptosis in human retinal pigment epithelial cells. Am J Ophthalmol 2004;137:931–933.
26 Barranger E, Grahek D, Cortez A, Talbot JN, Uzan S, Darai E: Laparoscopic sentinel lymph node procedure using a combination of patent blue and radioisotope in women with cervical carcinoma. Cancer 2003;97:3003–3009.
27 Rodrigues EB, Maia M, Meyer CH, Penha FM, Dib E, Farah ME: Vital dyes for chromovitrectomy. Curr Opin Ophthalmol 2007;18:179–187.
28 Westermeier R: Sensitive, quantitative, and fast modifications for Coomassie blue staining of polyacrylamide gels. Proteomics 2006;6:61–64.
29 Orgül S, Prünte C, Kain HL: Modellexperimente zur äusseren Blut-Retina-Schranke in vitro. Ophthalmologe 1992;89:400–404.
30 Mennel S, Peter S, Meyer CH, Thumann G: Effect of photodynamic therapy on the function of the outer blood-retinal barrier in an in vitro model. Graefes Arch Clin Exp Ophthalmol 2006;244:1015–1021.
31 Hartnett ME, Lappas A, Darland D, McColm JR, Lovejoy S, D'Amore PA: Retinal pigment epithelium and endothelial cell interaction causes retinal pigment epithelial barrier dysfunction via a soluble VEGF-dependent mechanism. Exp Eye Res 2003;77:593–599.
32 Mennel S, Thumann G, Peter S, Meyer CH, Kroll P: Influence of vital dyes on the function of the outer blood-retinal barrier in vitro. Klin Monatsbl Augenheilkd 2006;223:568–576.
33 Dunn KC, Aotaki-Keen AE, Putkey FR, Hjelmeland LM: ARPE-19, a human retinal pigment epithelial cell line with differentiated properties. Exp Eye Res 1996;62:155–169.
34 Orgul S, Reuter U, Kain HL: Osmotic stress in an in vitro model of the outer blood-retinal barrier. Ger J Ophthalmol 1993;2:436–443.
35 Hiebl W, Gunther B, Meinert H: Substances for staining biological tissues: use of dyes in ophthalmology. Klin Monatsbl Augenheilkd 2005;222:309–311.
36 Luke C, Luke M, Dietlein TS, Hueber A, Jordan J, Sickel W, Kirchhof B: Retinal tolerance to dyes. Br J Ophthalmol 2005;89:1188–1191.
37 Luke C, Luke M, Sickel W, Schneider T: Effects of patent blue on human retinal function. Graefes Arch Clin Exp Ophthalmol 2006;244:1188–1190.
38 Maia M, Penha F, Rodrigues EB, Principe A, Dib E, Meyer CH, Freymuller E, Moraes N, Farah ME: Effects of subretinal injection of patent blue and trypan blue in rabbits. Curr Eye Res 2007;32:309–317.
39 Hisatomi T, Enaida H, Matsumoto H, Kagimoto T, Ueno A, Hata Y, Kubota T, Goto Y, Ishibashi T: Staining ability and biocompatibility of brilliant blue G: preclinical study of brilliant blue G as an adjunct for capsular staining. Arch Ophthalmol 2006;124:514–519.
40 Enaida H, Hisatomi T, Goto Y, Hata Y, Ueno A, Miura M, Kubota T, Ishibashi T: Preclinical investigation of internal limiting membrane staining and peeling using intravitreal brilliant blue G. Retina 2006;26:623–630.
41 Ueno A, Hisatomi T, Enaida H, Kagimoto T, Mochizuki Y, Goto Y, Kubota T, Hata Y, Ishibashi T: Biocompatibility of brilliant blue G in a rat model of subretinal injection. Retina 2007;27:499–504.
42 Enaida H, Hisatomi T, Hata Y, Ueno A, Goto Y, Yamada T, Kubota T, Ishibashi T: Brilliant blue G selectivelpy stains the internal limiting membrane/brilliant blue G-assisted membrane peeling. Retina 2006;26:631–636.

PD Dr. Stefan Mennel
Department of Ophthalmology, Philipps-University Marburg
Robert-Koch-Strasse 4
DE–35037 Marburg (Germany)
Tel. +49 6421 889 528, Fax +49 6421 286 5678, E-Mail stefan.mennel@lycos.com

Meyer CH (ed): Vital Dyes in Vitreoretinal Surgery.
Dev Ophthalmol. Basel, Karger, 2008, vol 42, pp 115–125

Brilliant Blue in Vitreoretinal Surgery

Hiroshi Enaida[a,b] · Tatsuro Ishibashi[a]

[a]Department of Ophthalmology, Graduate School of Medical Sciences, Kyushu University, and [b]Department of Ophthalmology, Clinical Research Institute, National Hospital Organization, Kyushu Medical Center, Fukuoka, Japan

Abstract

This paper reviews the preclinical effects of brilliant blue G (BBG) on the morphology and functions of the retina, and reports on a pilot study of BBG staining and subsequent peeling of the internal limiting membrane (ILM) during vitreoretinal surgery. BBG solution was injected into rat eyes and investigated using light microscopy and electron microscopy, terminal deoxynucleotidyl transferase-mediated dUTP nick end labeling staining, and electroretinography (ERG). No pathological changes were caused by the BBG intravitreous injection. Although electron microscopy revealed that high doses of BBG induced vacuolization in the inner retinal cells, there was no reduction in the amplitude of the ERG waves and no detectable toxic effects. In the primate eyes, the ILM was clearly visualized by BBG staining, and peeled off easily from the retina. In the clinical study, BBG improved visualization of the ILM, allowing peeling and surgery to be performed successfully on patients with various vitroretinal diseases. Improvement of postoperative visual acuity was obtained in most cases, and no adverse effects were observed postoperatively. In conclusion, BBG has low toxicity, high staining ability, and is easy to handle, making it a good candidate dye for visualizing vitreoretinal disease surgery without adverse effects.

The retinal internal limiting membrane (ILM) acts as a basement membrane for the Müller cells of the retina. Alterations in the structure of the retina due to cellular proliferation might cause distortion of the ILM, leading to the formation of epiretinal membrane (ERM) holes and macular holes (MHs). Removal of the ILM can successfully alleviate these vitreoretinal diseases; however, difficulties in the visualization of the almost translucent ILM can present technical challenges in this procedure. It is now widely recognized that without a surgical adjuvant it is difficult to remove the membranes due to the poor visibility of the ILM and ERM. The staining of the ILM is therefore a crucial development in surgery for such vitreoretinal diseases [1–4]. The development of indocyanine green (ICG) and trypan blue (TB) staining has greatly facilitated the peeling of the ILM and ERM in the treatment of

Table 1. Osmolarity of dye solutions

Solution	Osmolarity, mosm/kg H_2O
BBG (10 mg/ml)	310
BBG (1 mg/ml)	300
BBG (0.25 mg/ml)	299
ICG (5 mg/ml)	271
TB (1 mg/ml)	316
Control (vehicle)	298

The control solution is Opeguard®-MA (Senju Pharmaceutical Co. Ltd., Osaka, Japan).

various vitreoretinal diseases, and, as a result, this technique is now widely used by many surgeons [5–7]. However, numerous clinical and experimental reports have recently suggested that intravitreous injections of ICG and TB can cause retinal damage [8–25].

A dye with both satisfactory staining ability at low concentrations and minimal toxicity is required for effective membrane staining. We have screened various dyes focusing on their safety and ability to stain membranes in vitreoretinal surgery. From the results of our preliminary analysis, we selected brilliant blue G (BBG) as a potent candidate for ILM staining [26–29].

In this report, we introduce preclinical and clinical results of BBG staining in vitreoretinal surgery.

Characterization of the Brilliant Blue G Solution

BBG is a blue dye that is also known as acid blue 90 and Coomassie brilliant blue G. BBG has been used for protein staining in biological fields, as it binds nonspecifically to most proteins. However, the pharmacological function of the dye remains unconfirmed. There have been no reports on the medical use of this dye with the exception of our previous study [29], although there is a long history of biological use with no apparent reported toxicity. The characterization of factors such as osmolarity of the solution is important in terms of cell survival [10, 25]. We therefore tested the osmo-

statistically significant differences between the amplitudes (**c**). Data are expressed as mean ± standard error of the mean of the amplitude compared with the control group.

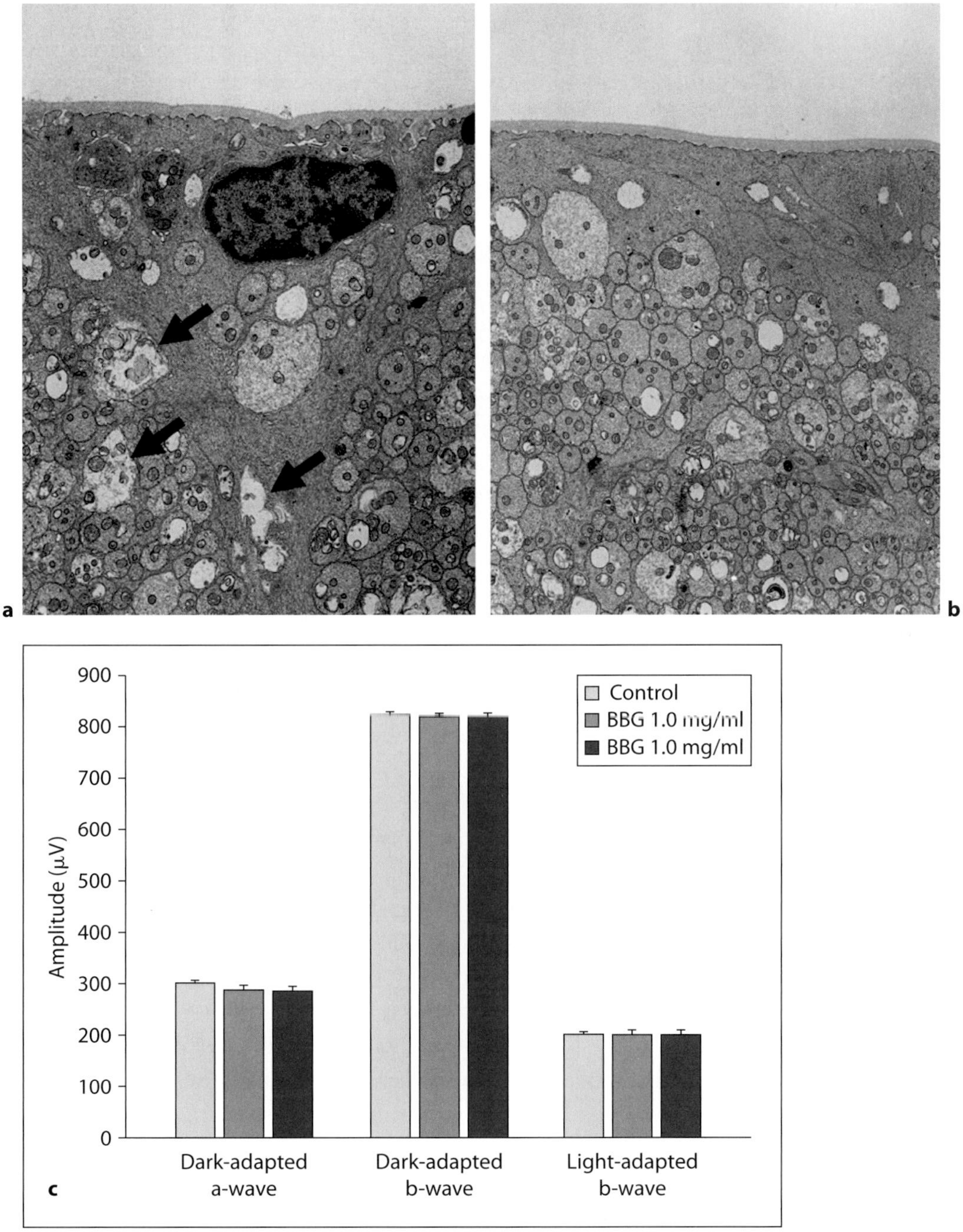

Fig. 1. TEM photography and maximal amplitudes of ERGs of rat eyes injected with intravitreous BBG (10 and 1 mg/ml; 0.05 ml/eye) visualized at 14 days. The highest-dose group (10 mg/ml) showed vacuolization in the ganglion cells and Müller cell processes of some specimens at day 14 (**a**). Although similar changes were also found in the 1 mg/ml group (**b**), the grade of vacuolization was less than that in the 10 mg/ml group (original magnification ×2,000). In the ERG examination, there was no reduction in the maximal amplitudes of the ERG waves in the high-dose groups, with no

larity of various concentrations of BBG, ICG, and TB solutions (table 1). ICG has a much lower osmolarity than the control, while that of TB is higher than the control value. By contrast, the osmolarity of BBG was found to be similar to those of intraocular irrigating solutions [26–28].

Preclinical Investigation of Brilliant Blue G for Internal Limiting Membrane Staining

All procedures conformed to the Association for Research in Vision and Ophthalmology Statement for the Use of Animals in Ophthalmic and Vision Research, and the Guidelines for Animal Care produced by Kyushu University, Fukuoka, Japan.

Effects of Intravitreous Injection of Brilliant Blue G in Rat Eyes

To investigate the effects of BBG on the morphology and functions of the retina, rat eyes were subjected to a gas compression vitrectomy, and various concentrations of BBG solution (10, 1, 0.1, and 0.01 mg/ml) were injected into the vitreous cavity. The eyes were enucleated at 2 weeks and 2 months. Light and transmission electron microscopy (TEM), terminal deoxynucleotidyl transferase-mediated dUTP nick end labeling (TUNEL) staining, and electroretinography (ERG) were used to investigate retinal damage and function [26].

In the rat eyes, no pathological changes were observed under light microscopy. TEM revealed that BBG at high doses (10 and 1 mg/ml) induced vacuolization in the ganglion cells and Müller cell processes. Vacuolization was not observed in the groups that received lower doses (0.1 and 0.01 mg/ml) or in the controls (fig. 1a, b). Among all groups, no remarkable changes were observed in the retina [including the inner nuclear, outer nuclear, and retinal pigment epithelial (RPE) cell layers] [26]. As there have been several recent reports regarding damage of the retinal cells caused by ICG and TB through apoptosis [16–21], we investigated apoptotic cell death using the TUNEL method. In the group injected with the highest doses of BBG (10 mg/ml), 1 case of apoptotic cell death was observed from among 10 sections. However, the apoptotic cell ratio was not significantly different to that observed in the control sections. In groups injected with lower doses of BBG, no TUNEL staining was observed in the retina [26].

To evaluate the retinal function after BBG injection, we performed ERG analysis in the high-dose groups (10 and 1 mg/ml). There was no reduction in the amplitude of the ERG waves in the high-dose groups compared with the control (fig. 1c).

After the intravitreous injection of BBG, no toxic effects (such as corneal edema, severe retinal edema, or endophthalmitis) were observed under surgical microscopy over a period of 2 months [26].

In our previous study, high doses (25 and 2.5 mg/ml) of intravitreous ICG were found to cause morphological damage in the rat retina when observed under light microscopy [8]. In groups injected with low doses (0.25 and 0.025 mg/ml), there was no apparent histological damage, but the amplitude of the dark-adapted (bipolar and Müller-cell-mediated) b-waves decreased in a dose-dependent manner, producing a significant difference compared to the controls [8]. High doses of intravitreous BBG injection did not cause retinal damage according to our examinations [26].

Effects of Subretinal Injection of Brilliant Blue G in Rat Eyes

To evaluate the toxicity of subretinal injections of BBG compared with ICG and TB, retinal detachments were produced by subretinal injections of the dyes. The biocompatibility of BBG (0.25 mg/ml) was evaluated over 2 months and 2 weeks by ophthalmic examinations. The eyes were enucleated, and analyzed by light and fluorescent microscopy, and TEM. Apoptotic cell death was detected by TUNEL staining. The results were compared with those of ICG (5 mg/ml) and TB (1 mg/ml) [28]. The final concentration of ICG and TB was determined according to the solution commonly reported in vitrectomies for humans [1–7].

ICG caused retinal degeneration and RPE cell atrophy 2 weeks after subretinal injection. Apoptotic cell death was detected in the inner and outer nuclear layers, and the RPE layer, especially in the photoreceptors. TB caused less retinal degeneration, which was mainly in the area detached by the subretinal injection. BBG had no detectable toxic effects after 2 months and 2 weeks. Apoptotic cell death was detected in the ICG and TB groups, mainly in the photoreceptors. Subretinal injection of the dyes caused retinal cell degeneration at lower concentrations than those reported for intravitreous injection. However, subretinal injection of BBG at a dose of 0.25 mg/ml appeared to provide satisfactory biocompatibility (fig. 2) [28].

Brilliant-Blue-G-Assisted Internal Limiting Membrane Peeling and Postoperative Examinations in Primate Eyes

As peeling of the ILM is impossible in rat eyes, we examined the ability of BBG to stain the ILM in primate eyes. After injecting 0.5 mg/ml BBG solution into the primate eyes, the ILM instantly stained light blue and was clearly visible. We were then able to easily remove the ILM with a forceps. Fluorescein angiography on day 14 also demonstrated that there was no apparent damage to the retina of the primate eyes.

Further ophthalmoscopic examinations showed no further changes in the retina during the 6-month follow-up period [26].

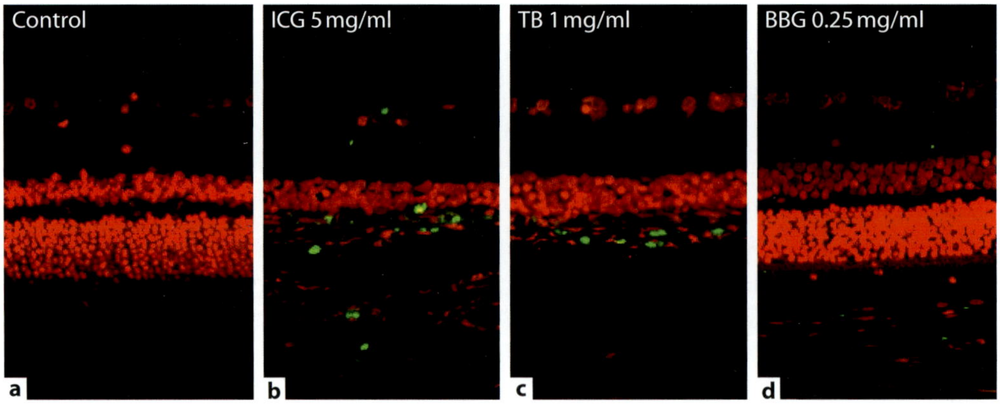

Fig. 2. Apoptotic cell death of rat eyes with dyes injected into the subretinal space as detected by TUNEL staining. ICG (**b**) and TB (**c**) showed TUNEL-positive apoptotic cell death mainly in the outer layers of the retinal and RPE cells. In the BBG group (**d**), no TUNEL staining was observed in the retinal or RPE cells (original magnification ×200).

Clinical Investigation of Brilliant Blue G for Internal Limiting Membrane Staining

This pilot study was carried out with approval from the Institutional Review Board, and performed in accordance with the ethical standards of the 1989 Declaration of Helsinki. The possible advantages and risks of the present treatment were explained to all of the patients before surgery, and written informed consent was obtained.

Pilot Study of Brilliant-Blue-G-Assisted Membrane Peeling

We investigated the staining patterns of membranes and the clinical outcomes using BBG in surgery for various vitreoretinal diseases.

BBG was dissolved in intraocular irrigating solution, and sterilized through a syringe filter to a final concentration of 0.25 mg/ml (pH 7.4). The prepared BBG solution was then injected gently into the vitreous cavity, and washed out immediately with balanced salt solution [29]. In cases of MHs, the ILM instantly stained light blue. Removal of the ILM was performed using a forceps (fig. 3a). Following the removal of the ILM, a difference in the retinal surface color between the area from which the ILM had been removed and the surrounding area was clearly visible (fig. 3b). In cases of diabetic macular edema, BBG solution was injected and washed out immediately after creating the posterior vitreous detachment, and the removal of the stained ILM was performed as easily as in the MH cases (fig. 3c). In the ERM cases, however, staining of the ERM could not be confirmed at this concentration.

After ERM peeling (fig. 3d, e), BBG solution was injected again, followed by immediate irrigation of the vitreous cavity. The ILM of the area where the ERM had been removed was strongly stained with BBG. However, the area where the residual ERM and posterior vitreous remained was not stained. The well-stained ILM could be easily removed (fig. 3f).

At a BBG concentration of 0.25 mg/ml, an accidental leakage into the subretinal space is predicted to have little influence on the retinal tissue [27]. Thus, for cases such as rhegmatogenous retinal detachment accompanied by an MH, for example, we used 0.25 mg/ml of BBG for ILM peeling (fig. 3g, h).

BBG also has a number of advantages over both ICG and TB in terms of handling. ICG is packaged as lyophilized powder, and will not dissolve in intraocular irrigating solution alone; BBG granules, by contrast, can be easily dissolved in intraocular irrigating solution alone, and can subsequently be sterilized with a 0.22-μm syringe filter. The osmolarity and pH value of the BBG solution are also stable [26–29]. Furthermore, the staining process requires no additional techniques, such as the fluid-air exchange that is necessary for TB application. The ILM staining pattern produced by the BBG solution was similar to that of the ICG solution, and, as BBG is not a fluorescence dye, there is little possibility of light toxicity such as that produced with ICG. In addition, the BBG concentrations required for staining the ILM are about 1/10–1/20 lower than that of ICG.

We have performed vitreous surgery using BBG for over 300 cases of various vitreoretinal diseases. More than 92% of these cases had their visual acuity preserved or improved, and no adverse effects were noted during the postoperative observation period.

From these studies, we can conclude that BBG is a potentially useful dye for ILM staining, and BBG-assisted membrane peeling is a potentially effective and safe means of managing vitreoretinal surgery. The safety of BBG in humans is not yet fully established. Further investigations are necessary before any clinical recommendation can be given.

Pharmacological Effects of Brilliant Blue G as a Possible Therapeutic Agent

BBG is a potent antagonist to purinergic nucleotide receptors ($P2X_7$). In the adult rat retina, $P2X_7$ was detected in the inner nuclear layer and the ganglion cell layer [30]. In the monkey retina, this receptor was observed in the inner nuclear layer, inner plexiform layer, and ganglion cell layer [31]. However, the function of $P2X_7$ has yet to be fully clarified. We used $P2X_7$ knockout (KO) mice to perform morphological and functional examinations. KO mice were obtained from Pfizer (Groton, Conn., USA) and breeds from Taconic (Germantown, N.Y., USA). Their corresponding wild type is C57BL/6J. No pathological differences were observed between $P2X_7$ KO mice and wild-type mice at 4, 10, and 40 weeks after birth. To evaluate the retinal function of $P2X_7$ KO mice, we also performed ERG analysis in both groups ($P2X_7$ KO and wild-type

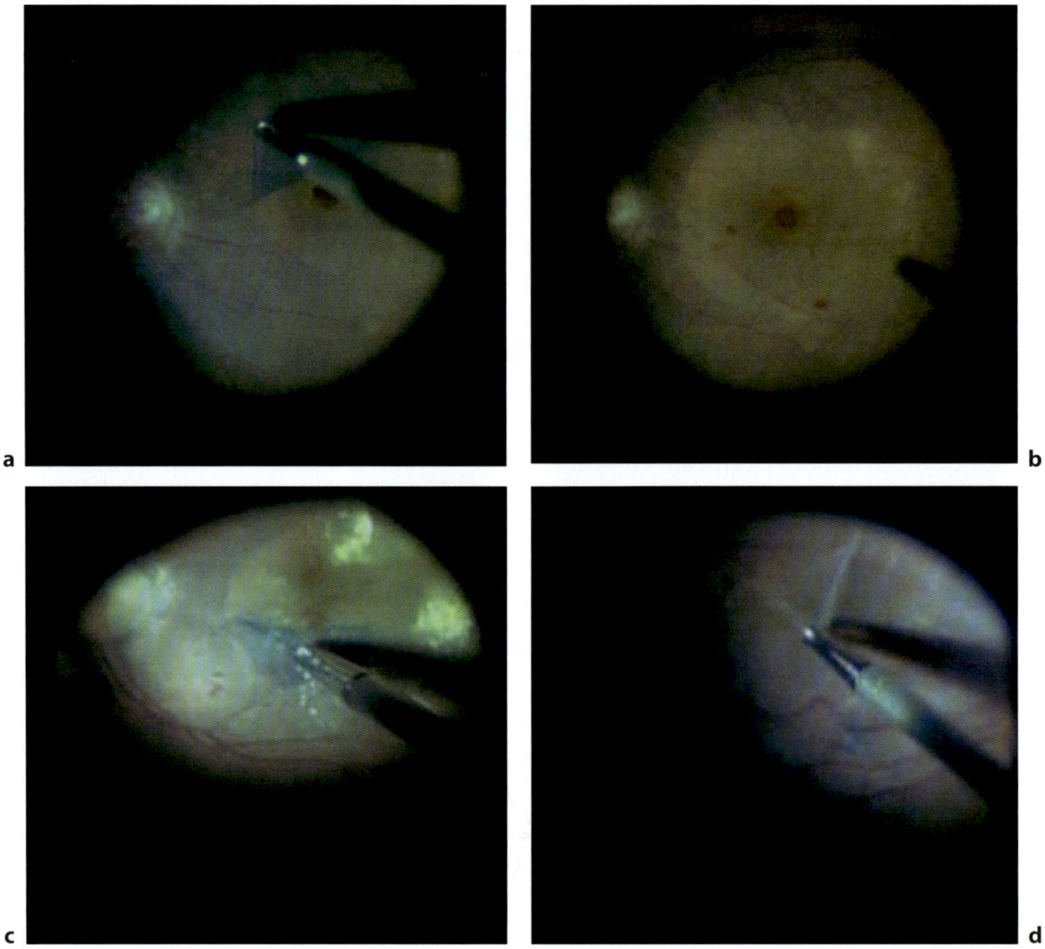

Fig. 3. BBG-assisted ILM peeling for various vitreoretinal diseases. **a** In MH cases, the ILM instantly stained light blue. The edge and flap of the ILM were clearly visible during ILM peeling. **b** Following the removal of the ILM, a difference in color of the retinal surface between the area from which the ILM had been removed and the surrounding area was clearly visible. **c** In diabetic macular edema cases, removal of the stained ILM was as easily performed as in MH cases. **d, e** Staining of the ERM could not be confirmed at this concentration. After peeling of the ERM, BBG solution was injected again and the vitreous cavity was irrigated immediately. The residual ILM of the area from which the ERM had been removed was strongly stained. **f** The strongly stained ILM was easily removed. **g, h** In cases such as rhegmatogenous retinal detachment accompanied by an MH, the ILM was peeled using 0.25 mg/ml BBG.

mice). There was no reduction in the amplitude of the ERG waves in either group (data not shown), and no adverse effects were observed in our examinations. Moreover, previous reports suggested that BBG suppresses retinal ganglion cell death [32], and inhibits phosphorylation of Src on the TNF-activated microglia [33]. Furthermore, according to the results of our study, BBG inhibits the growth of Müller

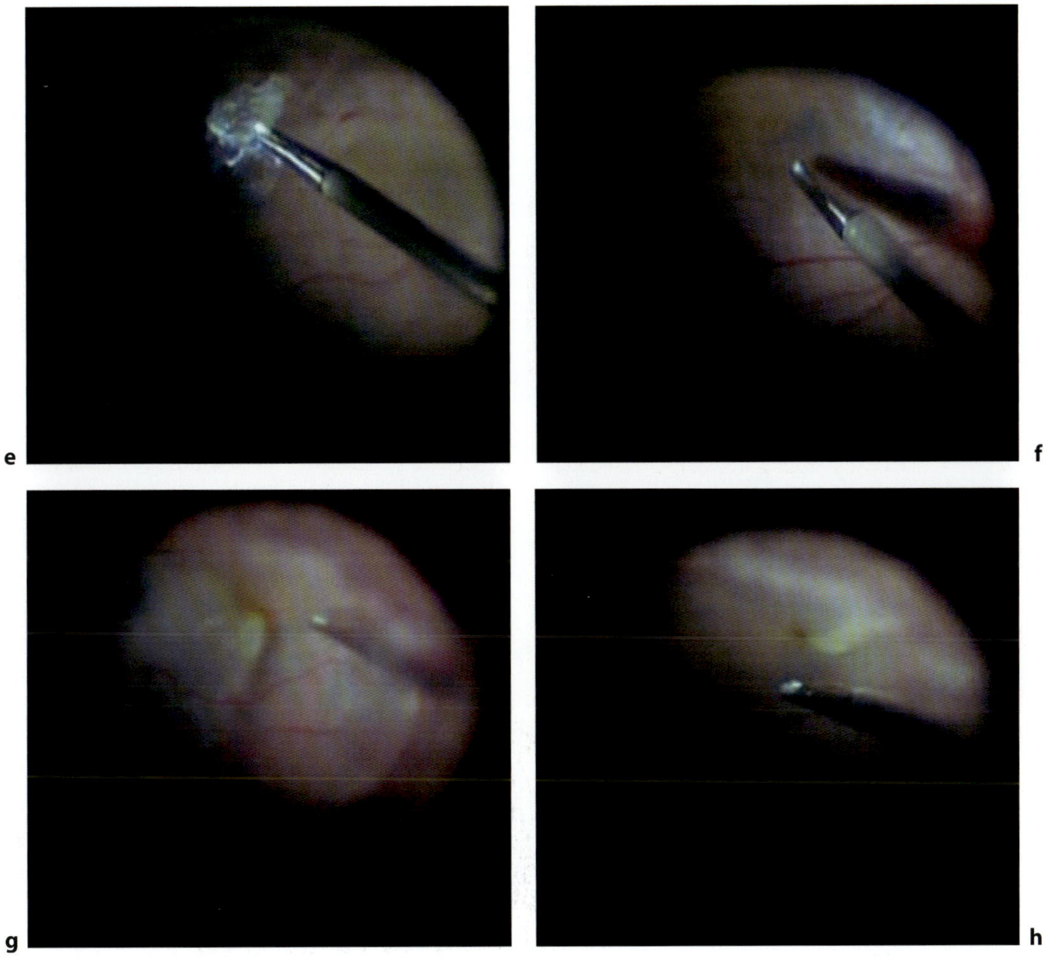

cells in vitro, which might be due to the blockade of the $P2X_7$ receptor. However, the exact mechanistic details remain to be investigated [34]. Since 0.25 mg/ml of BBG in addition to staining the ILM also inhibits cell proliferation, it might also offer postoperative benefits by reducing fibrous formation.

We are currently running clinical trials of BBG in parallel with further examinations to highlight its possible use as a therapeutic agent for surgery in various vitreoretinal diseases.

Acknowledgements

This work was supported in part by grant-in-aids No. 18591925 for Scientific Research from the Japanese Ministry of Education, Science, Sports and Culture and The Eye Research Foundation for the Aged.

References

1 Burk SE, Da Mata AP, Snyder ME, Rosa RH Jr, Foster RE: Indocyanine green-assisted peeling of the retinal internal limiting membrane. Ophthalmology 2000; 107:2010–2014.

2 Kadonosono K, Itoh N, Uchio E, Nakamura S, Ohno S: Staining of internal limiting membrane in macular hole surgery. Arch Ophthalmol 2000;118: 1116–1118.

3 Feron EJ, Veckeneer M, Parys-Van Ginderdeuren R, Van Lommel A, Melles GR, Stalmans P: Trypan blue staining of epiretinal membranes in proliferative vitreoretinopathy. Arch Ophthalmol 2002;120:141–144.

4 Perrier M, Sebag M: Trypan blue-assisted peeling of the internal limiting membrane during macular hole surgery. Am J Ophthalmol 2003;135:903–905.

5 Gandorfer A, Messmer EM, Ulbig MW, Kampik A: Indocyanine green selectively stains the internal limiting membrane. Am J Ophthalmol 2001;131:387–388.

6 Kusaka S, Hayashi N, Ohji M, Hayashi A, Kamei M, Tano Y: Indocyanine green facilitates removal of epiretinal and internal limiting membranes in myopic eyes with retinal detachment. Am J Ophthalmol 2001;131:388–390.

7 Haritoglou C, Eibl K, Schaumberger M, Mueller AJ, Priglinger S, Alge C, Kampik A: Functional outcome after trypan blue-assisted vitrectomy for macular pucker: a prospective, randomized, comparative trial. Am J Ophthalmol 2004;138:1–5.

8 Enaida H, Sakamoto T, Hisatomi T, Goto Y, Ishibashi T: Morphological and functional damage of the retina caused by intravitreous indocyanine green in rat eyes. Graefes Arch Clin Exp Ophthalmol 2002; 240:209–213.

9 Sippy BD, Engelbrecht NE, Hubbard GB, Moriarty SE, Jiang S, Aaberg TM Jr, Aaberg TM Sr, Grossniklaus HE, Sternberg P Jr: Indocyanine green effect on cultured human retinal pigment epithelial cells: implication for macular hole surgery. Am J Ophthalmol 2001;132:433–435.

10 Stalmans P, Van Aken EH, Veckeneer M, Feron EJ, Stalmans I: Toxic effect of indocyanine green on retinal pigment epithelium related to osmotic effects of the solvent. Am J Ophthalmol 2002;134: 282–285.

11 Gandorfer A, Haritoglou C, Gass CA, Ulbig MW, Kampik A: Indocyanine green-assisted peeling of the internal limiting membrane may cause retinal damage. Am J Ophthalmol 2001;132:431–433.

12 Haritoglou C, Gandorfer A, Gass CA, Schaumberger M, Ulbig MW, Kampik A: Indocyanine green-assisted peeling of the internal limiting membrane in macular hole surgery affects visual outcome: a clinicopathologic correlation. Am J Ophthalmol 2002; 134:836–841.

13 Uemura A, Kanda S, Sakamoto Y, Kita H: Visual field defects after uneventful vitrectomy for epiretinal membrane with indocyanine green-assisted internal limiting membrane peeling. Am J Ophthalmol 2003; 136:252–257.

14 Veckeneer M, van Overdam K, Monzer J, Kobuch K, van Marle W, Spekreijse H, van Meurs J: Ocular toxicity study of trypan blue injected into the vitreous cavity of rabbit eyes. Graefes Arch Clin Exp Ophthalmol 2001;239:698–704.

15 Haritoglou C, Gandorfer A, Schaumberger M, Priglinger SG, Mueller AJ, Gass CA, Kampik A: Trypan blue in macular pucker surgery: an evaluation of histology and functional outcome. Retina 2004;24:582–590.

16 Yam HF, Kwok AK, Chan KP, Lai TY, Chu KY, Lam DS, Pang CP: Effect of indocyanine green and illumination on gene expression in human retinal pigment epithelial cells. Invest Ophthalmol Vis Sci 2003;44:370–377.

17 Kawaji T, Hirata A, Inomata Y, Koga T, Tanihara H: Morphological damage in rabbit retina caused by subretinal injection of indocyanine green. Graefes Arch Clin Exp Ophthalmol 2004;242:158–164.

18 Rezai KA, Farrokh-Siar L, Ernest JT, van Seventer GA: Indocyanine green induces apoptosis in human retinal pigment epithelial cells. Am J Ophthalmol 2004;137:931–933.

19 Murata M, Shimizu S, Horiuchi S, Sato S: The effect of indocyanine green on cultured retinal glial cells. Retina 2005;25:75–80.

20 Rezai KA, Farrokh-Siar L, Gasyna EM, Ernest JT: Trypan blue induces apoptosis in human retinal pigment epithelial cells. Am J Ophthalmol 2004; 138:492–495.

21 Kwok AK, Yeung CK, Lai TY, Chan KP, Pang CP: Effects of trypan blue on cell viability and gene expression in human retinal pigment epithelial cells. Br J Ophthalmol 2004;88:1590–1594.

22 Ferencz M, Somfai GM, Farkas A, Kovacs I, Lesch B, Recsan Z, Nemes J, Salacz G: Functional assessment of the possible toxicity of indocyanine green dye in macular hole surgery. Am J Ophthalmol 2006; 142:765–770.

23 Saikia P, Maisch T, Kobuch K, Jackson TL, Baumler W, Szeimies RM, Gabel VP, Hillenkamp J: Safety testing of indocyanine green in an ex vivo porcine retina model. Invest Ophthalmol Vis Sci 2006;47: 4998–5003.

24 Maia M, Penha F, Rodrigues EB, Principe A, Dib E, Meyer CH, Freymuller E, Moraes N, Farah ME: Effects of subretinal injection of patent blue and trypan blue in rabbits. Curr Eye Res 2007;32:309–317.

25 Penha FM, Maia M, Eid Farah M, Principe AH, Freymuller EH, Maia A, Magalhaes O Jr, Smith RL: Effects of subretinal injections of indocyanine green, trypan blue, and glucose in rabbit eyes. Ophthalmology 2007;114:899–908.
26 Enaida H, Hisatomi T, Goto Y, Hata Y, Ueno A, Miura M, Kubota T, Ishibashi T: Preclinical investigation of internal limiting membrane peeling and staining using intravitreal brilliant blue G. Retina 2006;26:623–630.
27 Hisatomi T, Enaida H, Matsumoto H, Kagimoto T, Ueno A, Nakamura T, Hata Y, Kubota T, Goto Y, Ishibashi T: The biocompatibility of brilliant blue G: preclinical study of brilliant blue G as an adjunct for capsular staining. Arch Ophthalmol 2006;124: 514–519.
28 Ueno A, Hisatomi T, Enaida H, Kagimoto T, Mochizuki Y, Goto Y, Kubota T, Hata Y, Ishibashi T: Biocompatibility of brilliant blue G in a rat model of subretinal injection. Retina 2006;27:499–504.
29 Enaida H, Hisatomi T, Hata Y, Ueno A, Goto Y, Yamada T, Kubota T, Ishibashi T: Brilliant blue G selectively stains the internal limiting membrane/brilliant blue G-assisted membrane peeling. Retina 2006;26:631–636.
30 Brandle U, Kohler K, Wheeler-Schilling TH: Expression of the $P2X_7$-receptor subunit in neurons of the rat retina. Brain Res Mol Brain Res 1998;62: 106–109.
31 Ishii K, Kaneda M, Li H, Rockland KS, Hashikawa T: Neuron-specific distribution of $P2X_7$ purinergic receptors in the monkey retina. J Comp Neurol 2003; 459:267–277.
32 Zhang X, Zhang M, Laties AM, Mitchell CH: Stimulation of $P2X_7$ receptors elevates Ca^{2+} and kills retinal ganglion cells. Invest Ophthalmol Vis Sci 2005;46: 2183–2191.
33 Suzuki T, Hide I, Ido K, Kohsaka S, Inoue K, Nakata Y: Production and release of neuroprotective tumor necrosis factor by $P2X_7$ receptor-activated microglia. J Neurosci 2004;24:1–7.
34 Kawahara S, Hata Y, Miura M, Kita T, Sengoku A, Nakao S, Mochizuki Y, Enaida H, Ueno A, Moghadam AH, Ishibashi T: Intracellular events in retinal glial cells exposed to ICG and BBG. Invest Ophthalmol Vis Sci 2007;48:4426–4432.

Tatsuro Ishibashi, MD
Department of Ophthalmology, Graduate School of Medical Sciences, Kyushu University
3-1-1 Maidashi, Higashi-ku
Fukuoka, 812-8582 (Japan)
Tel. +81 92 642 5648, Fax +81 92 642 5663, E-Mail ishi@eye.med.kyushu-u.ac.jp

Meyer CH (ed): Vital Dyes in Vitreoretinal Surgery.
Dev Ophthalmol. Basel, Karger, 2008, vol 42, pp 126–140

Vital Staining and Retinal Detachment Surgery

Timothy L. Jackson

Department of Ophthalmology, King's College Hospital, London, UK

Abstract

The detection of retinal breaks is a key step in retinal detachment surgery. This chapter considers how vital stains might be used to enhance retinal break detection. Acid, basic, and neutral chromophores were used in the late 1930s and occasionally thereafter, but there are few reports on vital staining in the era of pars plana vitrectomy. One recent clinical study used a 41-gauge cannula to inject trypan blue into the subretinal space, in cases where no break could be identified by internal search. Heavy liquids were then used to vent the dye out of previously unseen retinal breaks, facilitating break detection. Laboratory studies of chromophores show that the degree and pattern of retinal staining depends on the characteristics of the chromophore – some dyes produce a linear, concentration-dependent increase in staining, others produce stepwise increments. Furthermore, the apparent hue of a dye may change with concentration and this may alter the color contrast with the predominantly red-orange background of the human fundus. Future studies may use fluorophore-tagged laboratory reagents to identify specific ocular tissues such as glia, interphotoreceptor matrix, retinal pigment epithelium, and devitalized tissue. These highly specific agents may facilitate vitreoretinal interventions other than retinal detachment surgery and there are many potentially exciting lines of inquiry.

Surgery for retinal detachment (RD) has improved markedly over the last 50 years, and the final reattachment rate continues to improve. By contrast, the success rate of primary RD repair has remained virtually static over the last 20 years. This is despite important technological advances such as the widespread introduction of pars plana vitrectomy, silicone oil tamponade, and wide-angle, noncontact, viewing systems. A study from Moorfields Eye Hospital in London compared results in 1973 with results in 1996 and found only a small, statistically nonsignificant improvement from 75 to 80% [1, 2]. Another study from St. Thomas' Hospital in London reported similar figures of 80 and 84% [3]. Results of a large national survey of RD surgery in the UK suggested that the primary success rate was only 82% (confidence interval 78–86%) amongst subspecialist vitreoretinal surgeons [4, 5]. Repeat surgery increases the inconvenience and anesthetic risks for the patient and is associated with serious complications such as proliferative vitreoretinopathy [6, 7] and a worse visual outcome [8, 9]. Patients who require more than one operation to reattach the retina also consume a disproportionately large amount of resources [10]. The low success rate of primary RD surgery, and importantly the failure to manifest any improvement in outcome, has been identified as an important deficit in vitreoretinal surgery [11, 12].

Analysis of why RD surgery fails indicates a number of causes including inadequate explant placement or retinopexy, traction from proliferative vitreoretinopathy, and new or missed breaks [2, 9, 13]. Of these, new or missed breaks may be the most important cause of failed primary RD surgery [2, 9]. It can be difficult to determine if the breaks responsible for failed surgery were present at the time of surgery and were missed by the surgeon, or occurred subsequently as new breaks. Some earlier studies suggest that the former are in the majority, accounting for 83% of this group [1]. It is difficult to confirm if this remains the case, but it is generally accepted that missed breaks remain an important cause of failed primary RD surgery [5]. There are also cases in which no break can be identified during RD surgery, a particularly challenging clinical situation. Finding retinal breaks is therefore an important and sometimes difficult requirement for successful RD repair.

This chapter considers previous attempts to enhance the detection of retinal breaks using vital stains, the limited recent literature on the subject, and strategies that might be explored in the future. Many of the potential targets for vital staining may be relevant not only to RD surgery, but also other vitreoretinal interventions. As such there are many exciting and unexplored lines of inquiry.

Historical Context

Despite the rapidly increasing number of reports on vital staining in macular surgery, there are, by comparison, far fewer reports on vital staining for RD surgery, and many of these were published more that 60 years ago. Chapter 3 offers some details of the history of ocular vital stains, including their use in RD, but key papers are also given in this chapter as they provide important background information on the suitability of certain types of dyes.

The first clinical report on vital staining for RD was by Sorsby, who also undertook a series of related animal experiments in the late 1930s [14–17]. Sorsby aimed to develop a systemically administered agent that could stain the retina *intra vitam*. The primary difficulty in achieving retinal staining was overcoming the blood-ocular barrier. Acid dyes such as trypan blue stained the retina but did not cross the blood-ocular barrier. By contrast, basic dyes such as methylene blue readily crossed the blood-ocular barrier but were lethal in most animals. The most satisfactory staining occurred with Kiton fast green, a basic dye with a sulfonate radicle. This agent was able to cross the blood-ocular barrier but the sulfonate group rendered the agent amphoteric and nontoxic. Preliminary experiments in rabbits showed that healthy retina did not stain, possibly due to conversion of the dye to its leukobase, whereas retina damaged by thermocautery stained green. Retina damaged by a septojod injection containing iodine and iodate also stained green. Sorsby made similar observations in a series of patients given the dye systemically. Chorioretinal lesions, and retinal and choroidal exudates were noted to stain with the dye whereas normal retina did not. Sorsby notes describes one patient with RD that 'illustrated the ease with which holes could be picked up in slightly stained detached retina' and that retinal holes were evident as red holes against this background staining.

In 1947, Black [18] repeated Sorsby's clinical studies investigating RD specifically. Patients received an intravenous injection of Kiton fast green, but he observed only a transient green flush of the arteries with no residual retinal staining. He discontinued the use of this dye because it produced prolonged staining of the patient's skin, and reported an alternative method using methylene blue. This was delivered via a transscleral route into the subretinal space. He reported that the choroid was unstained but detached retina stained blue. The primary aim was to make the RD easier to see. He noted that retinal tears were visible as red patches in bright contrast to the surrounding blue-stained retina. In addition, he observed that there were some reactive retinal pigment epithelium (RPE) changes suggestive of a 'mildly sclerosing action' when using a 1% solution. He felt that this might be helpful in maintaining retinal adhesion to the RPE but posed obvious risks with macula detachments.

In 1969, Kutschera [19] reported success using an intravitreal injection of disulfine blue in rabbits. Unlike the earlier papers, Kutchera administered the dye as an intravitreal injection with the specific aim of improving the detection of retinal breaks. Drawings show retinal breaks within areas of detached, lightly stained retina, but there was no specific staining of the retinal breaks themselves. Published clinical trials did not follow these experiments.

Chromophore Vital Stains

At present, nearly all reports on vital staining in ophthalmology are with chromophores. These agents function as biological stains and contain specific atomic groupings (C=S, C=N, N=N, N=O and NO_2) that are known to impart color [20]. These agents have the potential to enhance the color contrast of selectively stained ocular structures by absorbing and reflecting the illuminating light.

There are several classification systems for biological stains. One of the broadest divides compounds into natural or synthetic/artificial dyes [20]. However, this represents an unequal division as most available agents fall into the latter category. Historically, the chemical properties of a dye are more commonly used for classification, notably whether a dye is an acid, base or neutral.

The ideal chromophore would have several attributes: well-characterized binding; high tissue specificity; low cost; widespread availability, and clinical applicability, in particular a low potential for ocular or systemic toxicity. Acid chromophores may have an advantage as a dye to selectively stain retinal breaks as

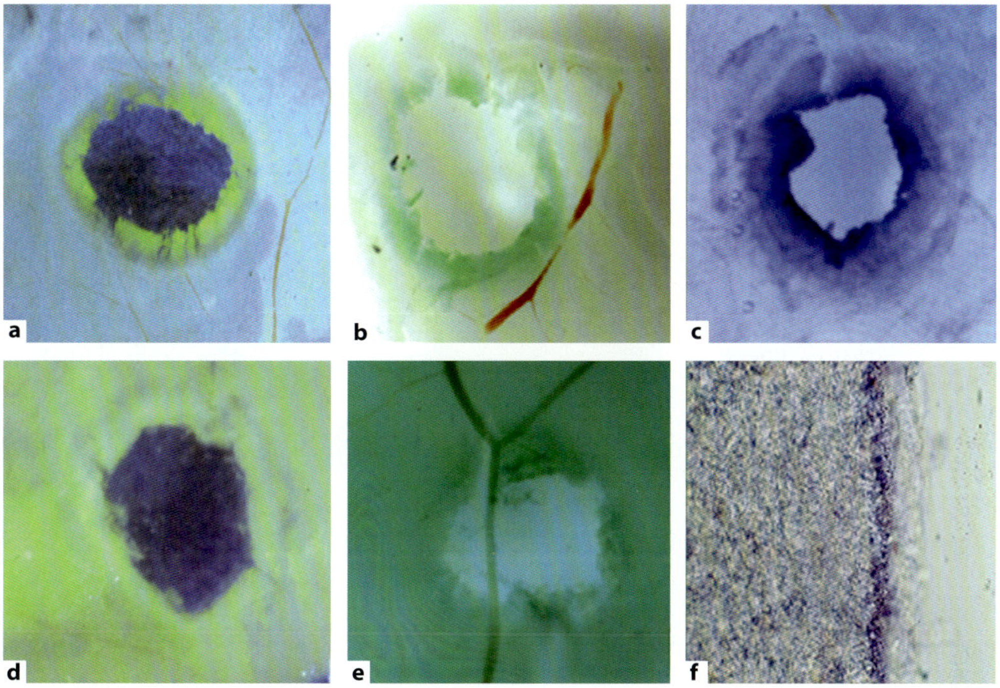

Fig. 1. Bovine retina stained with reactive yellow (**a, d**), fast green (**b, e**), and trypan blue (**c, f**). The holes visible in the upper panels were induced with the heated tip of a 20-gauge needle, with the flat mounts subsequently exposed to the vital stain. There is selective uptake of the dye by the damaged tissue at the margin of the break. When the retina was pretreated with methanol, all cells were devitalized, and subsequently reactive yellow and fast green stained all the tissue. **f** A flat mount exposed to trypan blue, without exposure to heat or methanol. The cut edge of the flat mount can be seen to stain blue; the mechanical cutting of the trephine causes devitalized tissue to take up the dye [22]. Taken together these images show that some dyes are able to selectively stain retinal tissue that has undergone mechanical, chemical, or heat damage.

they have an affinity for damaged neural tissue, are less likely to cross the blood-ocular barrier, and are generally safer than unmodified basic dyes [21].

Interestingly, many dyes stain damaged retinal tissue, whether the damage be mediated by mechanical tearing, heat, or chemical injury (fig. 1). Indeed, trypan blue is used in the laboratory to distinguish devitalized cells that take up the dye from healthy cells which do not (the so-called trypan blue exclusion test). It could therefore be predicted that fresh retinal tears might be selectively stained with a vital stain such as trypan blue.

Fluorophore Vital Stains

Fluorophores absorb light of one wavelength and then emit light of a longer wavelength. Indocyanine green was introduced as a fluorophore for use in choroidal

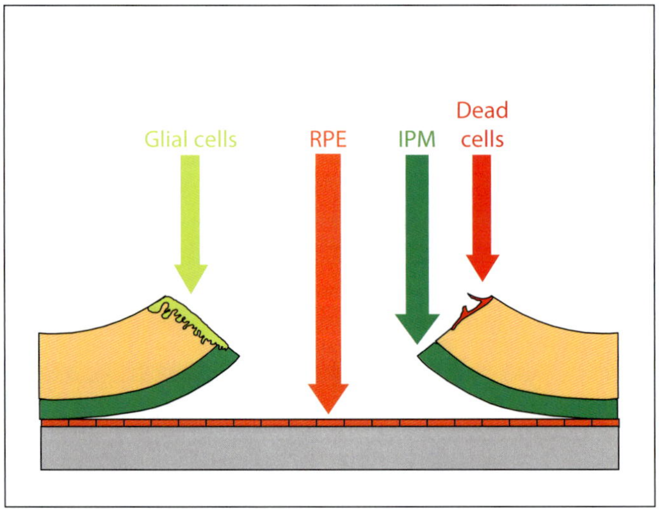

Fig. 2. A schematic diagram of a retinal break. The inner retinal surface is shown to the top of the upwardly convex retinal break. The vitreous cavity is shown in white, glial cells in yellow, RPE in orange, interphotoreceptor matrix (IPM) in green, and dead cells in red.

angiography but is applied as a chromophore when used as a macular vital stain. By use of selective optical filters it might be possible to selectively view structures that are stained with these agents, and proof of principle has been established [22]. Unlike most chromophores which appear to stain in a relatively nonspecific manner, the newer agents used in the laboratory for fluorescence microscopy have a much higher degree of tissue specificity, including antibodies that can be modulated to prevent complement binding and avoid a host inflammatory response. Therefore, antibodies, aptamers, and other histological agents with high tissue specificity might in the future be adapted for use as a surgical tool. This opens up the opportunity to target individual retinal structures, not only for the treatment of RD, but possibly for other surgical interventions.

Potential Targets

There are a number of potential targets for vital staining (fig. 2). Retinal breaks expose deep retinal structures such as the RPE and interphotoreceptor matrix (IPM) to the vitreous cavity. An intravitreal agent would therefore be able to selectively target these structures. Highly tissue-specific agents are available such as antibodies to the RPE, and lectins that target specific elements of the IPM. The shearing forces that result in a retinal break will cause tissue damage that might be stained by several dead-cell probes such as trypan blue. In addition, glial cells that traverse much of the retinal substrate will be exposed at the margin of the break. These could be targeted

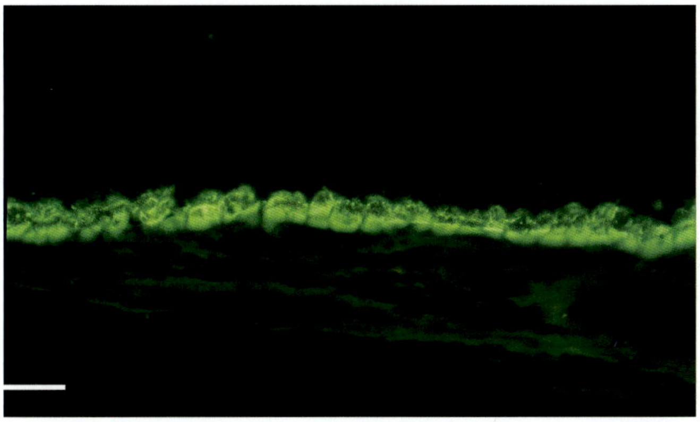

Fig. 3. A fluorescence photomicrograph of a bovine retina frozen section labelled with FITC-tagged anti-pancytokeratin (bar = 25 μm).

by glia-specific agents such as antibodies to glial fibrillary acidic protein (GFAP). The potential targets for staining are considered in turn.

Retinal Pigment Epithelium

A retinal break represents a discontinuity that exposes deep retinal and subretinal elements to the vitreous cavity. An intravitreal vital stain could therefore pass through this break to target these structures. Thus, one potential target is the RPE. Antibodies to RPE are available as shown in figure 3.

This strategy would be particularly useful for staining small breaks or holes in attached retina. In this setting, the vital stain would be expected to pass through the break, stain the underlying RPE, and thereby make the break more evident. However, it may have limited potential for staining retinal breaks within an area of detachment, as all of this area would be stained if any break were large enough to allow the dye to access the subretinal space. The ability to stain breaks in attached retina may have some clinical usefulness, but less than the ability to stain breaks in detached retina, as these are responsible for RD. The use of an RPE stain alone may therefore not be sufficient as an intraoperative vital stain.

Interphotoreceptor Matrix

The interphotoreceptor space exists between the external limiting membrane of the retina and the tight junctions of the RPE. This potential space is filled with the retinal IPM. The IPM is produced predominantly by the photoreceptors and may play a role in supporting metabolic function and mechanical attachment to the RPE. The soluble and insoluble constituents of the IPM are well characterized [23].

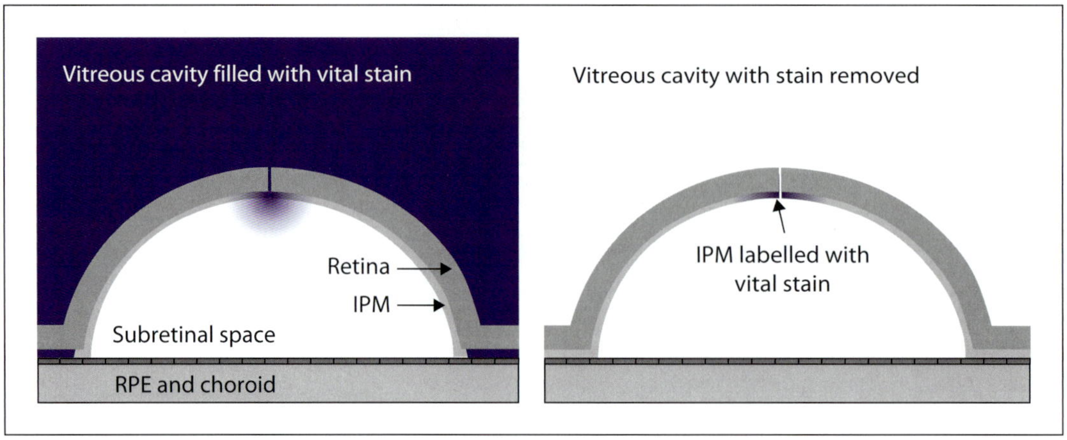

Fig. 4. A schematic drawing of an RD with a small retinal break at the apex. **a** The vitreous cavity filled with a vital stain directed at the IPM. **b** The postulated residual staining after the vital stain is rinsed from the vitreous cavity.

Targeting the IPM, like the RPE, has the disadvantage that it may potentially stain the entire inner retinal surface of detached retina. However, it is possible that this results in 'negative staining', if the retinal break or hole were seen as a nonfluorescent area against the background staining of the IPM. Conversely, it may be useful in the well-recognized situation in which a retinal break cannot be found during vitrectomy. In this setting, the break is invariably small and a vital stain would be particularly useful to the surgeon. An agent that targets the IPM might diffuse through this small break, selectively staining the IPM around the break, before becoming diluted in the subretinal fluid (fig. 4).

For these reasons, the IPM is a potentially more useful target than the RPE, and lectins are available to selectively target the IPM (fig. 5).

Three lectins are in common use in the laboratory: peanut agglutinin that binds the matrix surrounding cone apices; wheat germ agglutinin (derived from *Triticum vulgaris*) that binds the rod matrix, and *Helix aspersa* agglutinin that binds both.

Dead Cells

Acute retinal breaks, as opposed to atrophic retinal holes, are usually caused when the vitreous gel collapses and abnormal vitreoretinal adhesion creates a tear in the retina. This will produce an annulus of damaged tissue at the margin (edge) of the break. Agents are available that can stain dead and dying cells such as trypan blue. Many newer histological agents are available combined with fluorescent tags offering a higher degree of specificity. Some such as ethidium homodimer-1 enter damaged

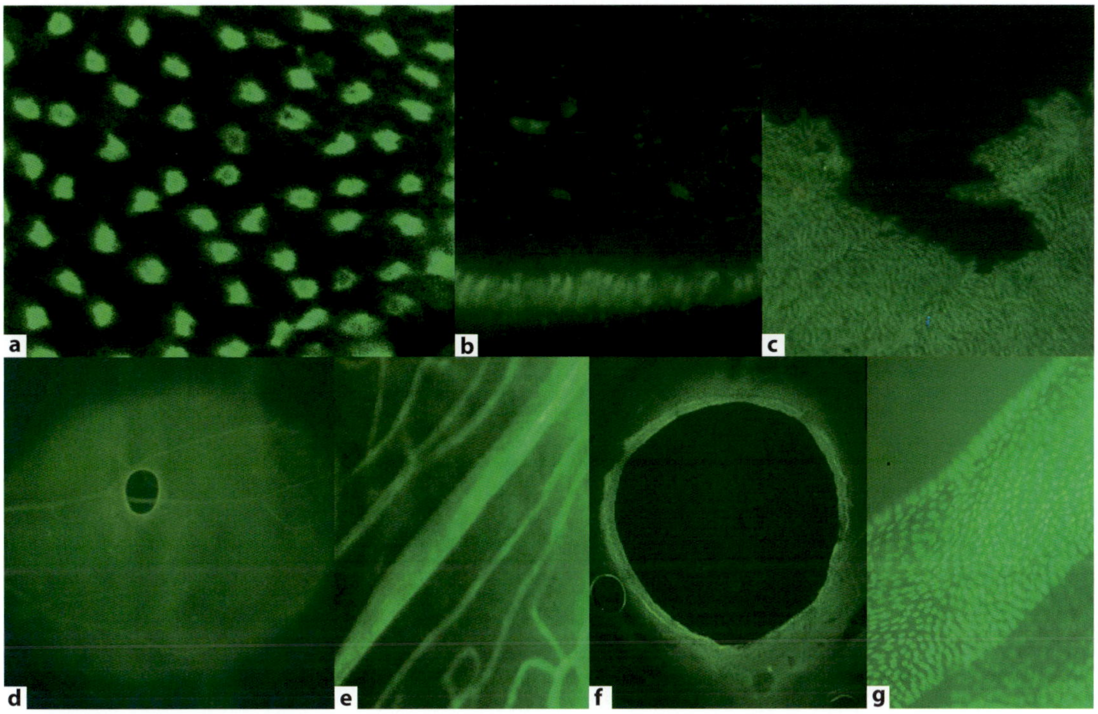

Fig. 5. Fluorescence microscope images of bovine retina stained with FITC-labelled lectins. **a** A flat mount viewed on the confocal microscope. **b** A frozen section. **c** A lower-power view of another flat mount, illustrating areas of nonstaining, presumably caused by denuded IPM. **d** Focal delivery to the retinal surface, but despite this there is some staining of vessels within the retinal substrate (**e**). The round, dark area within the brightly staining disk is an artifact from a bubble in the mounting media, and not a hole. **f** A retinal hole created with the tip of a 23-gauge needle, with increased fluorescence around its margin. A higher-power view (**g**) shows that this staining occurs at the upturned margin of the hole.

cells and bind to DNA, and have a bright fluorophore tag. Although this agent would not be appropriate because of potential toxicity, the principal of targeting devitalized tissue appears reasonable. The main weakness of this strategy is the fact that retinal breaks remodel, as indicated by experimental RDs in pig [24] and postmortem studies of human eyes [25–27]. This may limit the application of trypan blue or fluorophore markers to acute breaks, or those created at the time of surgery.

Intracellular Constituents

There are highly specific agents that can target intracellular filaments such as actin or tubulin, and it is possible that tearing of the cell walls at the margin of breaks may

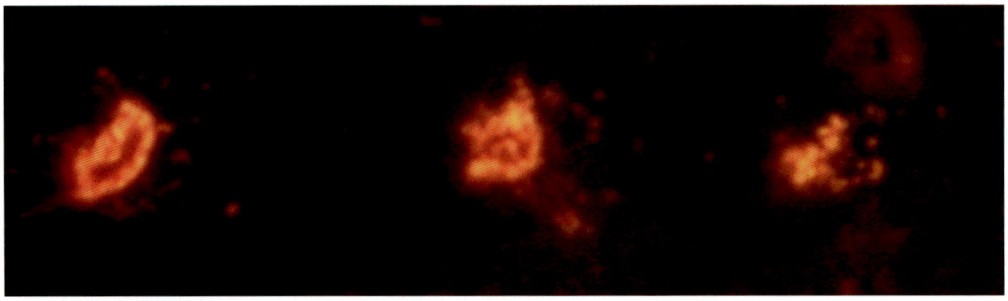

Fig. 6. Porcine retinal breaks created with needle puncture during pars plana vitrectomy, and then stained with intravitreal Cy3 anti-GFAP. Viewed under the microscope there is selective staining of the retinal breaks.

expose these intracellular constituents as a target for a vital staining. Of the intracellular constituents, the intermediate filaments of glial cells hold the most promise, as these are remarkably robust structures that can exist for extended periods outside the cell, and they can be selectively targeted with antibodies to GFAP. In the only study to date of fluorophore-assisted retinal break detection, Jackson and Marshall [22] used anti-GFAP to target the extruded glial filaments at the margin or retinal breaks in a pig model of detachment.

RDs were caused by creating a retinal break in a vitrectomized eye [24]. Laboratory grade anti-GFAP with a Cy3 fluorophore tag was exchanged using dialysis tubing into an intraocular saline solution. Once the animals had developed an RD, they were injected with anti-GFAP during a second vitrectomy. Using laser endoillumination with an emission spectrum that overlapped with Cy3 absorption, and barrier filters fitted to the operating microscope, it was possible to selectively view retinal breaks stained with anti-GFAP (figs. 6, 7). Ex vivo experiments showed that this staining occurred because the breaks disrupted the cell membrane but the tough intermediate filaments remained selectively stained. After 1 week, remodeling of the retinal break led to reduced staining, but the experiments did establish that fluorophore-assisted retinal break detection is possible.

Color Contrast and Dye Characteristics

The ideal retinal dye, either a chromophore or fluorophore, would provide good color contrast with unstained tissue. Therefore, blue/green dyes might show maximum contrast with the background yellow/orange hue of the human fundus. However, the clinical usefulness of this simplified approach is not known, and several factors may alter the color contrast and intensity of staining. As can be seen in figure 8, the apparent hue of a dye may change with concentration, and concentration of dye may vary

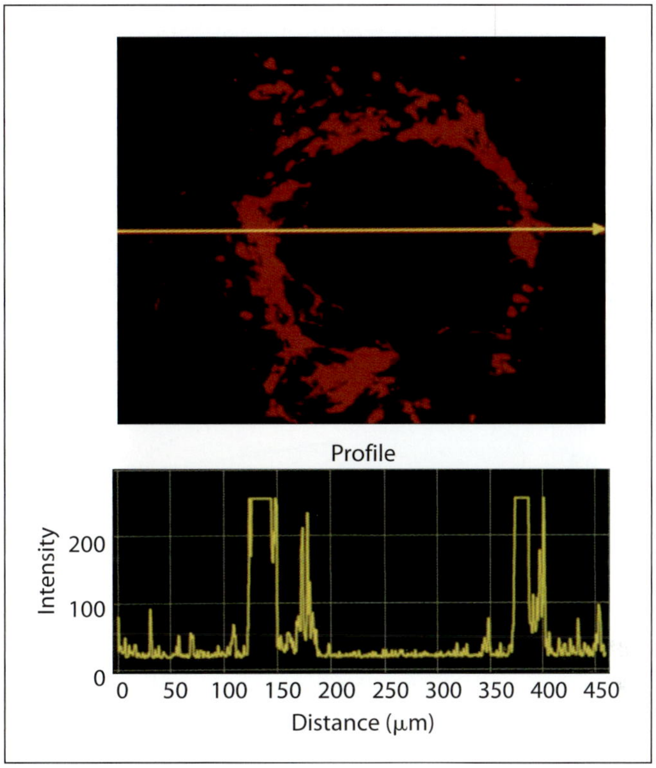

Fig. 7. A confocal image of an ex vivo, acute retinal break exposed to Cy3 anti-GFAP for 3 min. The Cy3 label can be seen to stain the intracellular filaments exposed in the cells at the margin of the break, creating selective staining of the break itself.

a

b

c

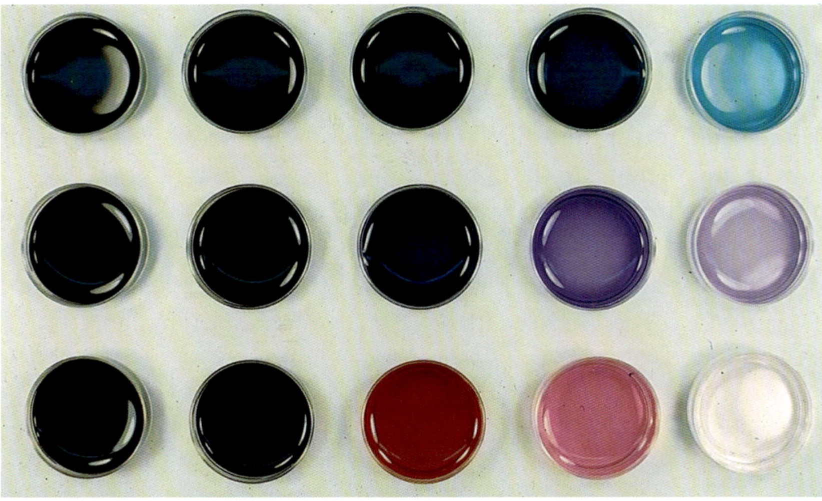

Fig. 8. Serial dilutions of fast green 10–0.01% (**a**), trypan blue 1–0.01% (**b**), and neutral red 2–0.002% (**c**).

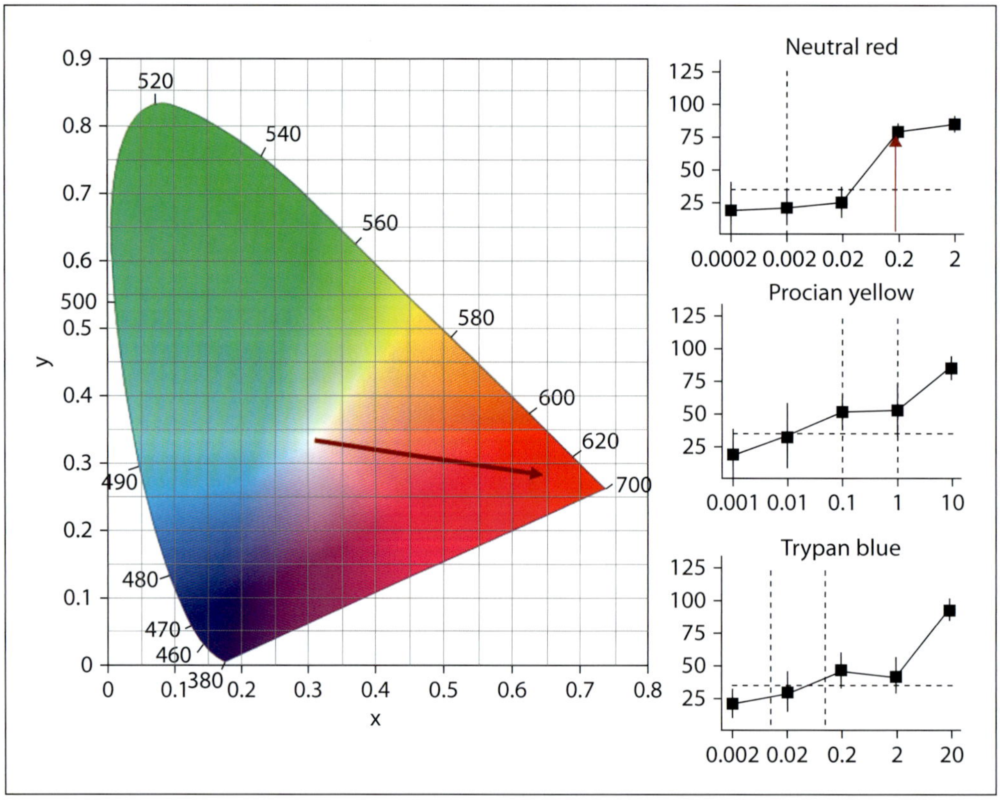

Fig. 9. The CIE 1931 color space chromaticity diagram, and the relationship between retinal staining and dye concentration in the three graphs on the right. By mapping unstained retina to a central white point, the magnitude of the color difference between this point and stained retina can be determined at a range of concentrations. As can be seen, dyes such as procian yellow show a roughly linear relationship between concentration (x-axis) and degree of staining (y-axis), whereas neutral red produces little staining until the concentration reaches 0.2%, at which point there is a large increase in color difference [28].

considerably if injected into a fluid-filled eye. Furthermore, the intensity of staining may not always be proportional to the concentration, as shown in figure 9.

In addition, not all retinal layers may stain uniformly. As figure 10 shows, some dyes produce a diffuse staining throughout the retinal substrate, whereas others tend to bind selectively to the inner retinal surface, when applied to this side. The uniformity of staining also varies with concentration, and between dyes, as shown in figure 11.

Subretinal Trypan Blue

The only clinical study of retinal vital staining in the vitrectomy era has recently been reported by Jackson et al. [29]. This study used subretinal trypan blue to identify

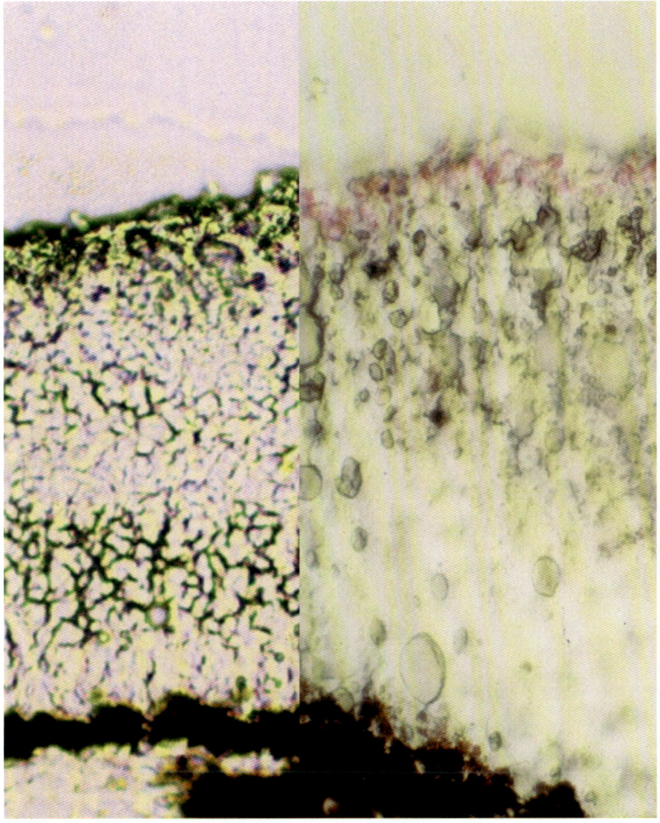

a b

Fig. 10. Frozen section of eyecups that had been partially filled with naphthol green (**a**) and Evans blue (**b**). Whereas naphthol green produced staining throughout the retinal substrate, Evans blue produced selective staining of the internal limiting membrane and possibly the inner nerve fiber layer [28].

retinal breaks in cases where no break could be found despite careful internal search. Cases where no retinal break can be identified during surgery represent a difficult clinical challenge, as failure to identify the break may lead to redetachment. It may mean that the surgeon has to use silicone oil, encircling explants, or extensive retinopexy, all of which can produce complications.

The authors used a 41-gauge silicone cannula designed for macular translocation surgery (fig. 12). This fine-bore cannula enabled them to introduce 0.15% trypan blue (Membrane Blue, DORC) into the subretinal space, without significant reflux through the puncture hole. Heavy liquid was then injected over the posterior pole, pushing the stained subretinal fluid out of the break. This produced a plume of dye that was visible to the surgeon from the previously unseen break (fig. 13).

This study modified a well-known technique that relies on the Schlieren phenomenon: proteinaceous subretinal fluid has a higher refractive index than the vitreous

a
b
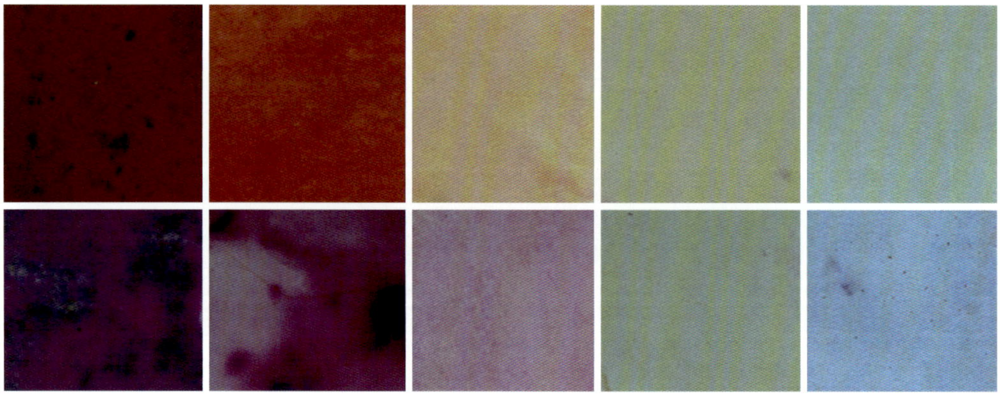

Fig. 11. Bovine retina exposed to serial dilutions of neutral red (**a**), and diethyloxadicarbocyanine (**b**). The concentration on the left is 2%, reduced by a factor of 10 with each dilution to 0.0002% at the far right. Neutral red appears to produce a relatively uniform uptake of dye except at the highest concentration, whereas even at low concentrations diethyloxadicarbocyanine produces sometimes patchy staining.

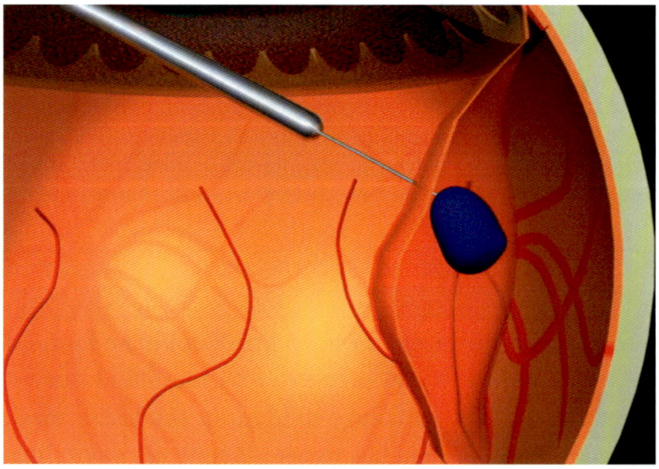

Fig. 12. Computer-generated image showing subretinal injection of trypan blue using a 41-gauge cannula (courtesy of G.W. Aylward).

infusate, and the subretinal fluid vented through a break by heavy liquid may be visible, and lead to detection of hard-to-find retinal breaks. By adding a subretinal dye, the contrast between the infusate and subretinal fluid was much more easily detected and in 4 of 5 cases the technique was successful. Even in the 1 case where no break

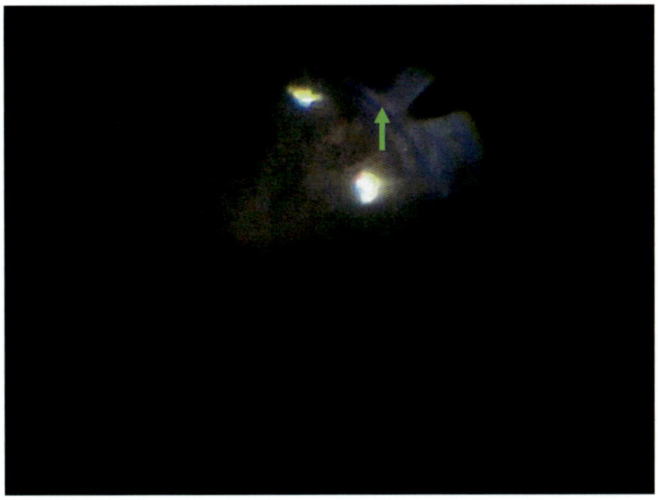

Fig. 13. Image capture of a video demonstrating the use of subretinal trypan blue to identify a retinal break [29]. A bubble of heavy liquid fills the eye up to the arrow, and just anterior to this the subretinal dye can be seen venting out of a previously unseen retinal break.

could be detected with trypan blue, the technique was helpful in excluding breaks in suspicious areas, thereby reducing the amount of cryotherapy applied.

Any potential toxicity was reduced by the heavy liquid that kept dye away from the fovea, and by rinsing dye from the subretinal space at the end of surgery using a drainage retinotomy. Although the puncture site from the 41-gauge cannula did not in theory require retinopexy, in some cases retinopexy was applied to ensure it did not subsequently cause an RD. It was noted that the dye is commonly applied to the fovea during macular hole surgery without manifest toxicity, but nonetheless the authors suggested that the technique was reserved for cases where no break could be detected, and not for routine use.

Interestingly, one break was detected when stained by trypan blue, consistent with the ex vivo experiments described earlier, showing that this agent stains damaged tissue at the edge of experimental retinal breaks.

Conclusion

The inability to detect retinal breaks can prolong surgery, result in additional surgical interventions with the risk of complications, and directly lead to anatomical failure. In this setting, subretinal trypan blue has been shown to be a useful surgical adjunct. However, there are many other biological stains that might be suitable for RD surgery and the vast majority of these remain untested. Furthermore, the possibility of using fluorophore-tagged agents with high levels of tissue specificity may, in the future, enable vital stains to further enhance the outcome of RD surgery, and possibly other vitreoretinal interventions.

References

1 Chignell AH, Fison LG, Davies EWG, et al: Failure in retinal detachment surgery. Br J Ophthalmol 1973; 57:525–530.
2 Sullivan PM, Luff AJ, Aylward GW: Results of primary retinal reattachment surgery: a prospective audit. Eye 1997;11:869–871.
3 Minihan M, Tanner V, Williamson TH: Primary rhegmatogenous retinal detachment: 20 years of change. Br J Ophthalmol 2001;85:546–548.
4 Thompson JA, Snead MP, Billington BM, et al: National audit of the outcome of primary surgery for rhegmatogenous retinal detachment. 1. Sample and methods. Eye 2002;16:766–770.
5 Thompson JA, Snead MP, Billington BM, et al: National audit of the outcome of primary surgery for rhegmatogenous retinal detachment. 2. Clinical outcomes. Eye 2002;16:771–777.
6 Bonnet M: Clinical factors predisposing to massive proliferative vitreoretinopathy in rhegmatogenous retinal detachment. Ophthalmologica 1984;188: 148–152.
7 Cowley M, Conway BP, Campochiaro PA, et al: Clinical risk factors for proliferative vitreoretinopathy. Arch Ophthalmol 1999;107:1147–1151.
8 Tani P, Robertson DM, Langworthy R: Rhegmatogenous retinal detachment without macular involvement treated with scleral buckling. Am J Ophthalmol 1980;90:503.
9 Laidlaw DA, Clark B, Grey RH, Markham RH: Results of primary retinal detachment surgery: a prospective audit. Eye 1998;12:751.
10 McCormack P, Simcock PR, Charteris DG, Lavin MJ: Is surgery for proliferative vitreoretinopathy justifiable? Eye 1994;8:75–76.
11 Wong D, McGalliard J: Are we getting better at treating retinal detachment? Technology, referral pattern or primary care? Eye 1997;11:763–764.
12 Snead MP, Scott JD: Results of primary retinal detachment surgery: a prospective audit. Eye 1998;12: 750.
13 Sharma T, Challa JK, Ravishankar KV: Scleral buckling for retinal detachment. Predictors of anatomic failure. Retina 1994;14:338–343.
14 Sorsby A, Elkeles A, Goodhart GW, Morris IB: Experimental staining of the retina in life. Proc R Soc Med 1937;30:1271–1273.
15 Sorsby A: Two patients with vital staining of the fundi. Trans Ophthalmol Soc UK 1938;58:275.
16 Sorsby A: Vital staining of the fundus. Trans Ophthalmol Soc UK 1939;59:727–730.
17 Sorsby A: Vital staining of the retina: preliminary clinical note. Br J Ophthalmol 1939;23:20–24.
18 Black GW: Some aspects of the treatment of simple detachment of the retina, including vital staining of the retina by methylene blue. Trans Ophthalmol Soc UK 1947;67:313–322.
19 Kutschera E: Vital staining of the detached retina with retinal breaks (in German). Albrecht Von Graefes Arch Klin Exp Ophthalmol 1969;178:72–87.
20 Lillie RD: H.J. Conn's Biological Stains, ed 9. Baltimore, Williams and Wilkins, 1977.
21 Sorsby A, Wright AD, Elkeles A: Vital staining in brain surgery. A preliminary note. Proc R Soc Med 1942;36:137–144.
22 Jackson TL, Marshall J: Fluorophore-assisted retinal break detection using antibodies to glial fibrillary acidic protein. Invest Ophthalmol Vis Sci 2004; 45:993–1001.
23 Hageman GS, Johnson LV: Biochemical characterization of the major peanut-agglutinin-binding glycoproteins in vertebrate retinae. J Comp Neurol 1948;249:499–510.
24 Jackson TL, Hillenkamp J, Williamson TH, et al: An experimental model of rhegmatogenous retinal detachment: surgical results and glial cell response. Invest Ophthalmol Vis Sci 2003;44:4026–4034.
25 Foos RY: Postoral peripheral retinal tears. Ann Ophthalmol 1974;679–687.
26 Foos RY: Retinal holes. Am J Ophthalmol 1978;86: 354–358.
27 Foos RY: Retinal tears and lesser lesions of the peripheral retina in autopsy eyes. Am J Ophthalmol 1967;64:643–655.
28 Jackson TL, Griffin L, Vote B, et al: An experimental method for testing novel retinal vital stains. Exp Eye Res 2005;81:446–454.
29 Jackson TL, Kwan AS, Laidlaw AH, Aylward W: Identification of retinal breaks using subretinal trypan blue injection. Ophthalmology 2007;114:587–590.

Timothy L. Jackson
Department of Ophthalmology
King's College Hospital
London SE5 9RS (UK)
Tel. +44 20 3299 3385, Fax +44 20 3299 3738, E-Mail Gillian.Williams@kch.nhs.uk

Meyer CH (ed): Vital Dyes in Vitreoretinal Surgery.
Dev Ophthalmol. Basel, Karger, 2008, vol 42, pp 141–152

An Experimental Approach towards Novel Dyes for Intraocular Surgery

Christos Haritoglou · Frank Schüttauf ·
Arnd Gandorfer · Sebastian Thaler

Department of Ophthalmology, Ludwig-Maximilians-University, Munich, and
Department of Ophthalmology, Eberhard-Karls-Universität Tübingen,
Tübingen, Germany

Abstract

Chromovitrectomy represents a recent development in the field of vitreoretinal surgery. Several dyes are available for intraocular application with different staining characteristics. Before the intraoperative use in humans, new dyes need to be evaluated thoroughly in experimental in vivo and ex vivo studies in order to detect potential adverse effects related to dye toxicity. This article describes a reasonable approach for the assessment of novel dyes prior to the use in humans

Target Structures of Chromovitrectomy

The primary goal of dye-assisted vitrectomy (chromovitrectomy) is to make surgical procedures safer and easier, especially for the less experienced surgeon. Vital dyes facilitate vitreoretinal surgery by visualizing nearly transparent structures such as the internal limiting membrane (ILM), epiretinal membranes (ERMs) or the vitreous. Especially ILM peeling has become a widely used surgical technique for the treatment of traction maculopathies. However, ILM peeling represents a true challenge to the vitreoretinal surgeon, as this delicate structure is only a few micrometer thick. Therefore, effort was made to develop a technique to visualize the ILM. Thus, the ILM became the first target structure of 'chromovitrectomy'. As a consequence, staining of the ILM allowed even the less experienced surgeons to follow the principle of ILM peeling and opened the possibility to better functional and anatomic results of macular surgery. The introduction of vital dyes to assist vitreoretinal surgery was greeted with great enthusiasm as this difficult surgical maneuver suddenly appeared to be – at least in theory – easier, safer and more controlled.

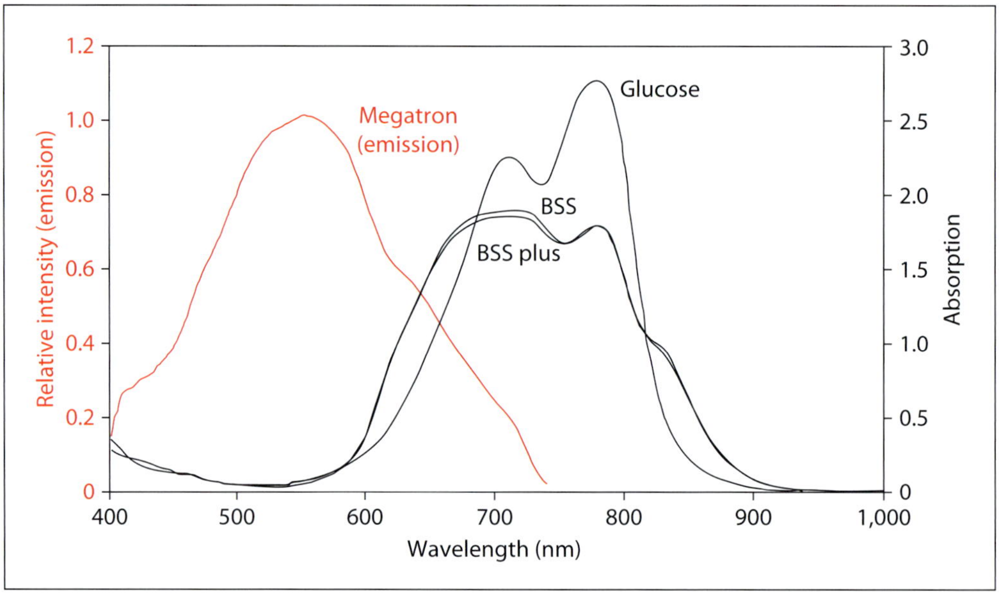

Fig. 1. Emission of the light source and absorption of different ICG solutions. The overlap between these curves may be the underlying mechanism for phototoxic properties of ICG solutions.

Among the first dyes introduced to stain the ILM was indocyanine green (ICG) during macular hole surgery [1, 2]. However, given the present controversial information in the literature [3–8], ICG became a subject of ongoing discussions and does not appear to be an ideal dye for intraocular use due to its narrow safety margin as indicated by clinical and experimental data suggesting some dye-related toxicity. As we do not completely understand the underlying mechanisms of action as well as the safety margins of ICG, its applicability seems to be limited. Indeed ICG is a very unstable dye when diluted in watery solutions and has photosensitizing properties (fig. 1). Another dye, trypan blue, was introduced to stain ERMs, without any signs of dye-related toxicity up to now [9, 10].

Besides staining of an ERM or the ILM, visualization of the vitreous itself has become a field of interest among vitreoretinal surgeons. The vitreous has been shown to function as a scaffold for fibrovascular proliferation [11]; interactions of vitreous collagen fibers and the innermost retina at the vitreoretinal interface represent the underlying mechanism of action for tractional vitreoretinal diseases. Therefore, the thorough removal of the vitreous and the posterior hyaloid membrane is an important goal during vitreoretinal procedures to treat macular holes, vitreoretinal traction syndrome, retinal detachment and many other conditions. Therefore, in addition to ERMs and the ILM, the staining and visualization of the vitreous seems to be an important aspect of 'chromovitrectomy' [12], a new field in vitreoretinal surgery.

Experimental Studies

It is beyond question that vital dyes being injected into the human eye need to be safe and potential toxic effects have to be ruled out in advance. (Of note, this had not been the case with ICG, which had been applied into the human eye without any preceding experimental studies addressing potential side effects of this off-label use.) Therefore, before the application in humans, all potential new dyes need to be carefully evaluated experimentally, both in in vivo and ex vivo settings. In what follows, the experimental investigation of potential new dyes for intraocular surgery is described as well as the first experiences in humans. The presented approach represents the personal experiences of our study group; different settings have been published in the literature [13].

Gross Evaluation of the Staining Properties ex vivo and Other Qualities

The evaluation of the staining properties of potential new dyes for intraocular surgery is quite a difficult task. As there are differences in the ocular anatomy between animals (primates and nonprimates) and humans, results obtained in animal studies cannot necessarily be transferred to the situation in humans. As a consequence, although as much safety data as possible should be obtained prior to the application in humans, the real value of a dye will become apparent following injection into the human eye. One might think of different models to get an impression of the staining properties of a dye. For example, one could choose to stain lens capsule material extracted from the eye during cataract surgery. Like the ILM, the lens capsule represents a true basement membrane of the eye. Epiretinal tissue removed during macular pucker or macular hole surgery could also be stained immediately after surgery. However, with this approach one will have difficulties in determining which surface of the membrane came into contact with the dye: the inner vitreal surface or the outer retinal surface. In addition, all dyes need to be checked for their photochemical stability, absorption spectrum and solubility in water.

However, using these techniques we were able to identify a number of novel candidates for intraocular application: light green SF yellowish (LG SF); E68; bromophenol blue (BPB); Chicago blue (CB); rhodamine 6G, and rhodulinrein blue 3G (basic blue 3). The dyes were then further evaluated concerning their toxicity in different experimental settings.

Evaluation of Staining Characteristics

The staining effect in removed lens capsule material and ERMs varied between the different dyes and dye concentrations applied. Using E68, BPB, CB, and rhodamine 6G resulted in pronounced staining of the lens capsule (fig. 2), whereas LG SF did not sufficiently stain the lens capsule using concentrations of 0.5% or less and only a concentration of 1% provided weak staining of ERMs. The other dyes revealed excellent

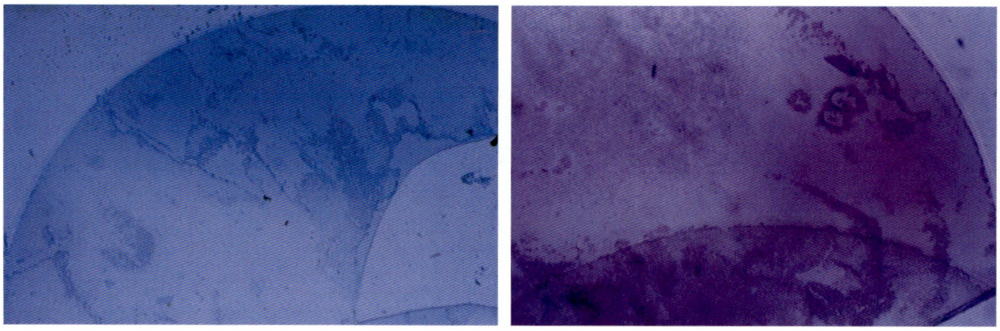

a b

Fig. 2. Staining of the lens capsule using CB (**a**) and BPB (**b**). The material was extracted during cataract surgery.

to good staining effects both in the lens capsule and ERMs even at a lower concentration of 0.2%. In porcine eyes, where the dye was poured over the anterior lens capsule in situ, the anterior lens capsule could be stained well with BPB, CB and E68, while LG SF provided weak staining effects.

Light-Absorbing Properties

Absorption spectra were obtained of 0.05% dye solutions. The light-absorbing properties and peaks of maximum absorption of dye concentrations of 0.05% were variable. The long wavelength maximum peak of absorption was in the range of 527–655 nm. Except for LG SF and rhodamine 6G, no dye showed relevant light absorption between 400 and 500 nm. Absorption maxima beyond 700 nm were not found for any of the investigated dyes (fig. 3).

Experimental Studies ex vivo (Cell Culture Models)

It seems of great importance to investigate novel dyes using different cell cultures. In our investigations, we chose ARPE-19 and primary RPE cells. This allowed for a stepwise assessment of dye-related toxicity. Dyes affecting cell survival of ARPE-19 cells were not further evaluated in primary RPE cell lines. Additionally, dyes showing toxic effects in cell cultures do not appear to be applicable in vivo and were therefore excluded from future investigations in animals. It seems reasonable to perform different tests to assess cell viability, such as the MTT assay and life-dead assays.

Evaluation of Dye Toxicity

MTT Assay. Compared to balanced salt solution plus (BSS plus) without addition of any dye serving as a control, 4 novel dyes (LG SF; E68; BPB, and CB) showed no significant impact on cell survival of ARPE-19 cells neither at a concentration of 0.2 nor 0.02%. Rhodamine G6 and rhodulinrein blue 3G revealed toxic effects at a concentra-

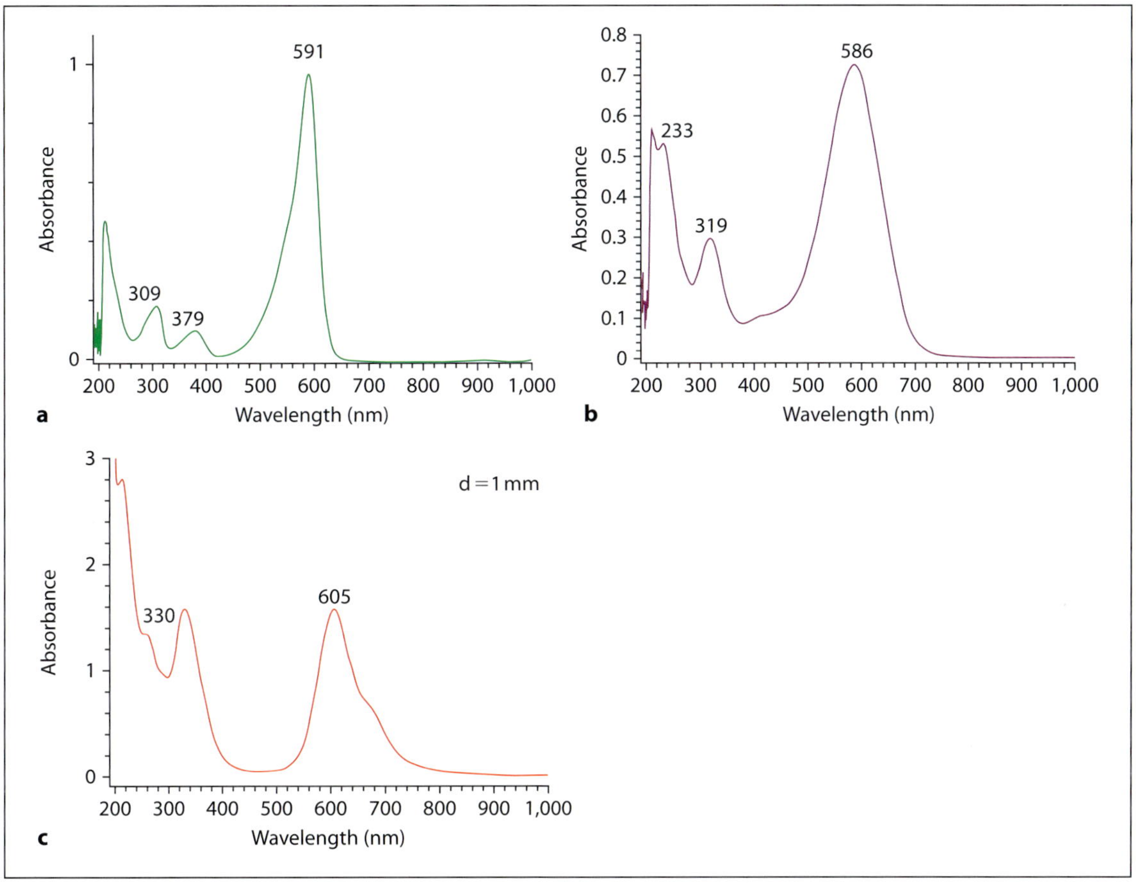

Fig. 3. Light absorption of the dyes investigated: BPB (**a**), CB (**b**), E68 (**c**).

tion of 0.2%, which was less severe at a concentration of 0.02%. Additionally, no influence on cell survival of primary RPE cells was observed after exposure to LG SF, E68, BPB and CB at concentrations of 0.2 and 0.02%. The differences between both concentrations were statistically significant only for rhodamine G6 ($p \leq 0.05$) in ARPE-19 cells and LG SF ($p \leq 0.05$) and ICG ($p \leq 0.05$) in primary RPE cells.

Life-Dead Assay. When the viability of RPE cells was tested by labeling of the nuclei of nonviable cells with propidium iodide 24 h after treatment of cells, 2 dyes (LG SF and CB) were identified to significantly affect cell viability compared to controls treated with BSS plus alone. After treatment with CB, this effect was seen both in cultures of ARPE-19 and primary RPE cells at concentrations of 0.2 and 0.02%. However, in comparison to the 0.2% dye solution, 0.02% LG SF appeared to be far less toxic. E68, BPB and BSS plus (control) did not affect cell survival.

Experimental Studies in vivo

Following the assessment of dye-related toxicity the dyes were further evaluated in vivo. These studies were performed to investigate potential long-term adverse effects. The total exposure time in these investigations was 7 days, a period of time being far longer than any potential exposure time during surgery in humans.

Long-Term Toxicity Studies
Rats were injected intravitreally with 4 dyes: LG SF, E68, BPB and CB dissolved in BSS at concentrations of 0.5 and 0.02%. BSS served as a control. Additional animals were treated with single injections of 0.5, 0.02, 0.002, and 0.0002% ICG or 0.002% E68 into one eye. Adverse effects on anterior and posterior segments were evaluated by slit lamp biomicroscopy and ophthalmoscopy. Retinal toxicity was assessed by histology and retinal ganglion cell quantification 7 days after dye administration.

Clinical Examination. Rat eyes were injected intravitreally with either dye or BSS plus without complications. No animal had to be excluded from further analysis due to difficulties related to intravitreal drug administration. Animals injected with either E68 0.5% or ICG 0.5% showed discrete staining of both the cornea and lens in the respective color of the dye. Staining was also present but to a clearly lesser extent in eyes injected with CB 0.5%. After injections with lower concentrations of the above-mentioned or other dyes, examination by slit lamp biomicroscopy showed no evidence of toxicity to the anterior segment of the eye such as corneal opacification or cataract induction. No visible inflammatory response in the form of vitreous opacification and/or retinal perfusion defects was seen with indirect ophthalmoscopy at any of the examination time points.

Histology. Qualitatively, the whole retina of eyes treated with BPB (0.5 and 0.02%), LG SF (0.5 and 0.02%) or the control BSS revealed normal morphology. The central retina also satisfied quantitative criteria for normal morphology.

Treatment with CB resulted in a heterogeneous incidence of morphological alterations. Of the 3 eyes treated with 0.5% CB, 1 eye showed no morphological alterations, 1 eye showed a focal mild loss of photoreceptors and loss of cells in the ganglion cell layer, and 1 eye showed an increase in hyalocytes in the vitreous. Of the 3 eyes treated with 0.02% CB, 2 were without morphological alterations, yet 1 eye showed focally complete outer retinal degeneration in the mid-peripheral region. Since this pathology lay outside the region of quantification, the measurements of the central retina showed normal values.

Treatment with E68 led to a consistently dose-dependent reaction. At a concentration of 0.5%, all eyes showed signs of inflammation with numerous leukocytes between the photoreceptor outer segments (mean number of leukocytes: 9.3 ± 1.8/mm); 1 eye also showed an accumulation of hyalocytes in the vitreous. The inflammation was pronounced in the middle and peripheral regions and less intense in the central region of the retina. A concentration of 0.02% still triggered leukocyte infiltrations (mean number of leukocytes: 3.7 ± 1.6/mm), but these were less numerous than in the group treated with 0.5% E68. At concentrations of 0.002 and 0.0002%, no morphological alterations were noted anywhere in the retina.

All eyes treated with 0.5% ICG showed degenerative changes. Quantification revealed a significant thinning of the inner retinal layers compared to BSS control eyes. Focal changes in the outer retina were also seen; these were located in the central and mid-peripheral regions. 0.02% ICG still resulted in focal changes in 2 out of 4 eyes. However, quantification of the different layers showed no statistically significant decrease. No morphological alterations of the retina were seen with lower concentrations of ICG (0.002 and 0.0002%).

Retinal Ganglion Cell Count. Seven days after intravitreal injections of E68 0.5% and ICG at all tested concentrations a significant loss of retinal ganglion cells was observed compared to BSS-injected control eyes. The most dramatic loss of ganglion cells was recorded after E68 0.5% injection, when the number of retinal ganglion cells dropped to 1,263 ± 195 cells/mm^2 (mean ± SEM, $p < 0.0001$). A less pronounced, but still significant loss of retinal ganglion cells was seen after ICG injections at 0.5% (2,197 ± 43; $p = 0.0254$), 0.02% (2,190 ± 56; $p = 0.0277$), 0.002% (2,141 ± 50; $p = 0.0116$) and 0.0002% (2,172 ± 65; $p = 0.0407$) (fig. 4). This finding may underline that ICG-related toxicity is not so much a question of the dye concentration but of other factors such as photosensitivity.

At the same time point, injections with lower concentrations of E68 or other dyes did not lead to statistically significant retinal ganglion cell loss. The BSS injection alone did not influence retinal ganglion cell survival compared to untreated eyes.

As a consequence of these investigations [14, 15], CB and BPB appear to be safe for application in humans.

Dye Application in Humans

Two dyes, BPB and CB, were used to assist vitreoretinal surgery and anterior segment surgery in humans following the above-mentioned experiments. The staining properties of CB are equal to trypan blue. Up to now, most clinical experience has been obtained with BPB (C19H10Br4O5S, FW 670), which was used in the past as a vital stain to probe the blood-brain barrier, as a protein stain and as a pH indicator [16].

Bromophenol Blue: Staining of the Epiretinal Membranes, Vitreous and Lens Capsule

BPB powder was dissolved and diluted using BSS plus and sterilized using a 0.22-μm syringe filter. A final dye concentration of 0.2% was then injected into the eye. We initially performed a core vitrectomy, followed by vitreous removal in the periphery in the area of the sclerotomy sites by indentation of the globe using a squint hook.

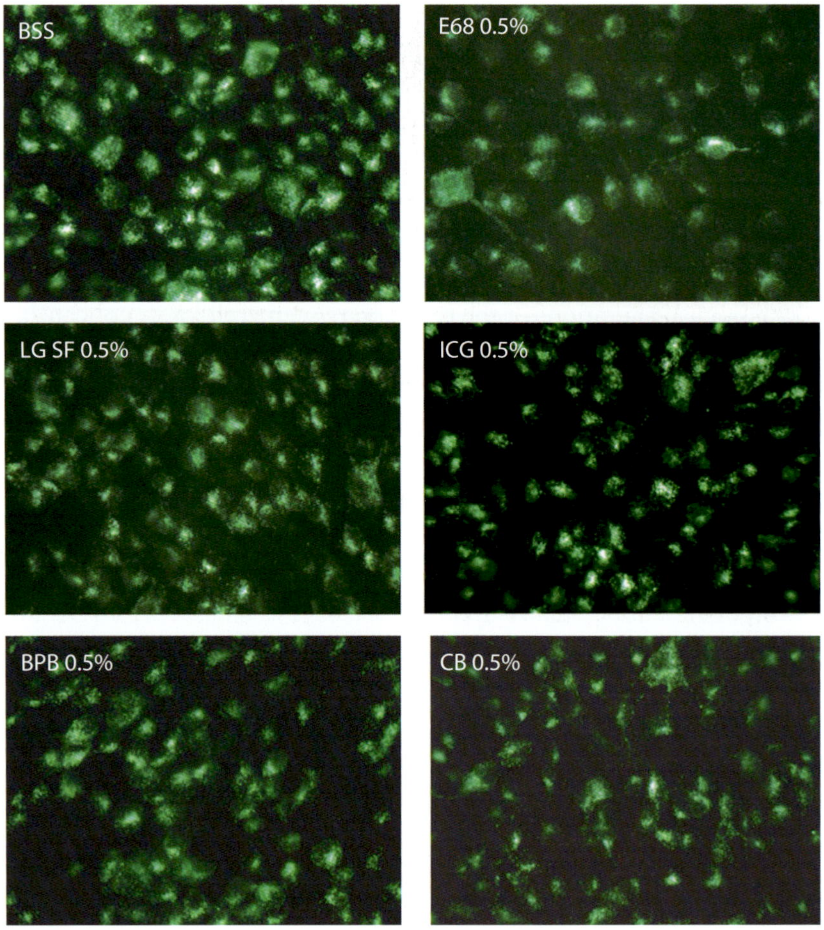

Fig. 4. Ganglion cell count in rat eyes.

We suggest different ways of dye application, depending on which structure the surgeon is aiming at. During pars plana vitrectomy for a macular hole a fluid-air exchange is performed prior to dye injection to achieve a maximum dye concentration on the retinal surface. Then, a few drops of the dye are injected over the posterior pole and the globe is gently moved to allow for an adequate dye distribution. This is followed by removal of excessive dye by irrigation after 1 min.

During surgery for retinal detachment one could apply the dye after induction of a posterior vitreous detachment and injection of approximately 1.5 ml heavy liquid and fluid-air exchange without removing the perfluorocarbon liquid in order to stain peripheral vitreous. Using this approach, one will not only obtain a higher dye concentration in the anterior segment of the eye as the dye cannot be further diluted by the perfluorocarbon liquid, but one could also prevent an uncontrolled distribution,

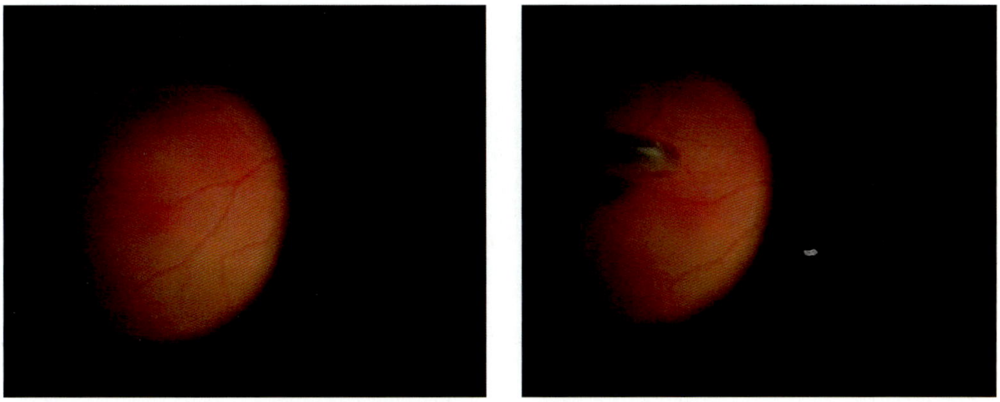

Fig. 5. Staining of a thin layer of attached posterior vitreous using BPB.

especially in the subretinal space, and excessive contact with the lens capsule, which may result in an unwanted staining effect. As a modification, one may inject the dye in the fluid-filled eye to stain posterior parts of the vitreous. An uncontrolled distribution in the subretinal space through retinal breaks could be prevented by partial fluid-air exchange and injection of the dye into the remaining fluid. In some conditions, one may also consider injecting the dye at the very beginning of surgery in order to achieve complete staining of the vitreous.

The dye was also used in the anterior segment to assist cataract surgery for mature cataracts; i.e., the dye was either injected into the air-filled anterior chamber and carefully removed by injection of viscoelastic material immediately after injection or injected after having filled the anterior chamber with viscoelastic material. In the latter case, the dye was evenly and gently distributed on the lens surface using a cannula and excessive dye was removed after completion of capsulorrhexis (approximately 1 min after application) [17–18].

Staining Effect and Clinical Implications

BPB appeared to be very useful to stain the adherent posterior hyaloid membrane and visualize interactions in terms of tractional forces of the vitreous on the retinal surface and in the macular area in macular hole patients with incomplete posterior vitreous detachment (fig. 5). Undetected remnants of an adherent posterior hyaloid membrane may contribute to anatomical failure of macular hole surgery, especially in lower-stage macular holes (II and III), where a complete detachment of the posterior hyaloid membrane is usually not seen. Thus, BPB may serve as a useful adjunct in macular hole surgery, especially for less experienced surgeons, as the dye helps to visualize both ERMs [18] and adherent vitreous cortex, and therefore allows a reliable induction of posterior vitreous detachment. This may be sufficient to successfully treat smaller macular holes as indicated by recent reports [19], and excessive ILM peeling may

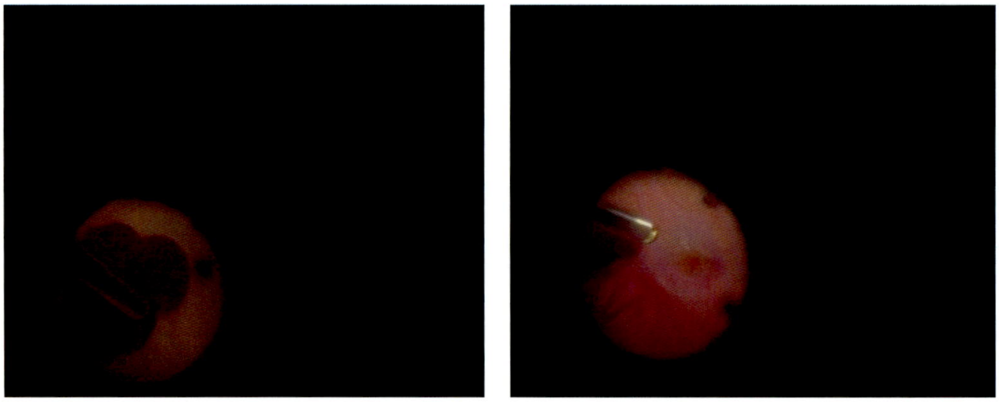

Fig. 6. Staining of an ERM using BPB.

consequently not be necessary. During pars plana vitrectomy for retinal detachment the visualization of the vitreous enables the surgeon to perform a complete removal of tractional forces, especially in the area of the retinal break and the vitreous base. This is relevant to prevent redetachments of the retina in the postoperative course, especially as the vitreous can serve as a scaffold for fibrovascular proliferation [11].

BPB was also very useful to stain and visualize ERMs (fig. 6). As described earlier, the dye was injected into the air-filled globe. The staining properties varied between patients. In patients with clinically visible ERMs satisfying staining of the membrane was noted. Less strong staining was noted in cases where it was difficult to remove ERMs or the ILM, suggesting that the pathological alterations were more pronounced within the retina and not on the retinal surface as seen in cases of classic ERMs. We did not observe sufficient staining of the ILM using this dye.

In the anterior segment, BPB allowed a predictable and uniform staining of the anterior lens capsule due to the direct contact of the dye with the capsule. An excellent contrast between the white lens and the stained lens capsule was noted in all patients, and the dye did not penetrate the lens capsule. There was no unwanted staining of other tissues such as the iris or the corneal endothelium.

Chicago Blue: Staining of the Epiretinal Membranes and Lens Capsule

CB was the second dye investigated in humans. CB is a large hydrophilic tetrasulfonated anionic dye and has been applied as a selective collagen stain in Masson trichrome and Van Gieson methods. In our experiments, the dye was used in concentrations of 0.1% to assist macular pucker surgery and cataract surgery. The dye helped to clearly stain ERMs and greatly facilitated their removal. All in all, the staining properties are equal to trypan blue in the posterior segment (fig. 7).

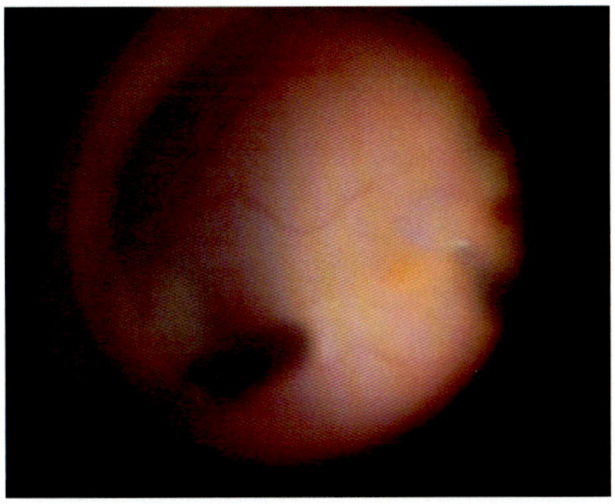

Fig. 7. Peeling of an ERM which was stained using CB.

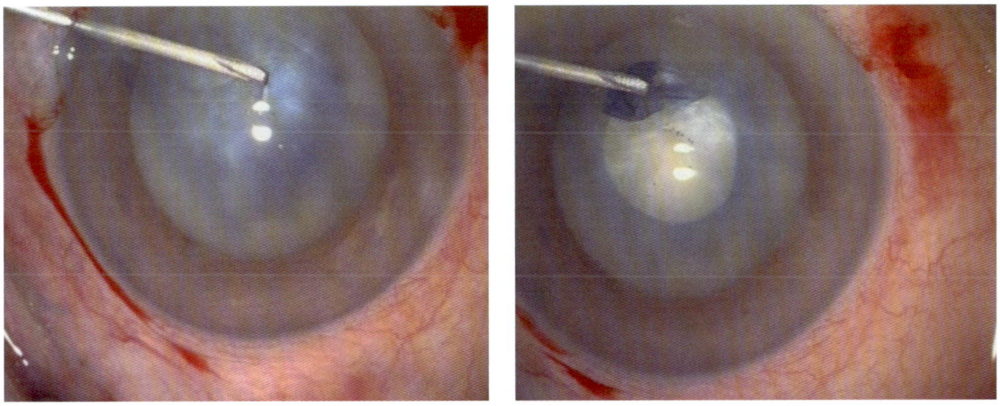

Fig. 8. Capsulorrhexis in a case of mature cataract using CB as a dye to stain the lens capsule.

In the anterior segment, the dye was used to assist surgery for mature cataracts. In all cases, a strong staining of the anterior lens capsule was seen (fig. 8).

We did not observe any negative effects we could attribute to the dye during our prospective investigations, which are still ongoing [data unpublished].

Conclusion

Chromovitrectomy is an emerging field in ophthalmology. Vital dyes may greatly facilitate certain surgical steps both during surgery in the anterior as well as in the posterior segment of the eye. A careful evaluation of the staining characteristics as well as of potential adverse effects is mandatory before the application of any dye in humans.

References

1 Yoshida M, Kishi S: Pathogenesis of macular hole recurrence and its prevention by internal limiting membrane peeling. Retina 2007;27:169–173.

2 Kadonosono K, Itoh N, Uchio E, et al: Staining of internal limiting membrane in macular hole surgery. Arch Ophthalmol 2000;118:1116–1118.

3 Tognetto D, Grandin R, Sanguinetti G, et al, Macular Hole Surgery Study Group: Internal limiting membrane removal during macular hole surgery: results of a multicenter retrospective study. Ophthalmology 2006;113:1401–1410.

4 Haritoglou C, Gandorfer A, Gass CA, et al: Indocyanine green-assisted peeling of the internal limiting membrane in macular hole surgery affects visual outcome: a clinicopathologic correlation. Am J Ophthalmol 2002;134:836–841.

5 Haritoglou C, Gandorfer A, Gass CA, et al: The effect of indocyanine-green on functional outcome of macular pucker surgery. Am J Ophthalmol 2003; 135:328–337.

6 Kanda S, Uemura A, Yamashita T, et al: Visual field defects after intravitreous administration of indocyanine green in macular hole surgery. Arch Ophthalmol 2004;122:1447–1451.

7 Burk SE, Da Mata AP, Snyder ME, et al: Indocyanine green-assisted peeling of the retinal internal limiting membrane. Ophthalmology 2000;107: 2010–2014.

8 Da Mata AP, Burk SE, Foster RE, et al: Long-term follow-up of indocyanine green-assisted peeling of the retinal internal limiting membrane during vitrectomy surgery for idiopathic macular hole repair. Ophthalmology 2004;111:2246–2253.

9 Haritoglou C, Gandorfer A, Schaumberger M, Priglinger SG, Mueller AJ, Gass CA, Kampik A: Trypan blue in macular pucker surgery: an evaluation of histology and functional outcome. Retina 2004;24: 582–590.

10 Feron EJ, Veckeneer M, Parys-Van Ginderdeuren R, Van Lommel A, Melles GRJ, Stalmans P: Trypan blue staining of epiretinal membranes in proliferative vitreoretinopathy. Arch Ophthalmol 2002;120: 141–144.

11 Nishimura M, Ikeda T, Ushiyama M, Kinoshita S, Yoshimura M: Changes in vitreous concentrations of human hepatocyte growth factor (hHGF) in proliferative diabetic retinopathy: implications for intraocular hHGF production. Clin Sci (Lond) 2000;98:9–14.

12 Rodrigues EB, Meyer CH, Kroll P: Chromovitrectomy: a new field in vitreoretinal surgery. Graefes Arch Clin Exp Ophthalmol 2005;243:291–293.

13 Haritoglou C, Yu A, Freyer W, et al: An evaluation of novel vital dyes for intraocular surgery. Invest Ophthalmol Vis Sci 2005;46:3315–3322.

14 Schuettauf F, Haritoglou C, May CA, et al: Administration of novel dyes for intraocular surgery: an in vivo toxicity animal study. Invest Ophthalmol Vis Sci 2006;47:3573–3578.

15 Horobin RW, Kiernan JA (eds): Conn's Biological Stains, ed 10. Oxford, BIOS Scientific Publishers Ltd, 2002, p 216.

16 Haritoglou C, Priglinger SG, Strauss R, Gandorfer A, Kampik A: Staining of the lens capsule during surgery for mature cataracts using bromphenol blue. J Cataract Refract Surg, in press.

17 Haritoglou C, Strauss R, Priglinger SG, Kreutzer T, Kampik A: Delineation of the vitreous and posterior hyaloid using bromphenol blue. Retina 2008;28: 333–339.

18 Haritoglou C, Schumann R, Strauss R, et al: Vitreoretinal surgery using bromphenol blue as a vital stain: evaluation of staining characteristics in humans. Br J Ophthalmol 2007;91:1125–1128.

19 Tadayoni R, Gaudric A, Haouchine B, Massin P: Relationship between macular hole size and the potential benefit of internal limiting membrane peeling. Br J Ophthalmol 2006;90:1239–1241.

Christos Haritoglou, MD
Department of Ophthalmology, Ludwig-Maximilians-University
Mathildenstrasse 8
DE–80336 Munich (Germany)
Tel. +49 89 5160 3811, Fax +49 89 5160 5160, E-Mail christos.haritoglou@med.uni-muenchen.de

Meyer CH (ed): Vital Dyes in Vitreoretinal Surgery.
Dev Ophthalmol. Basel, Karger, 2008, vol 42, pp 153–159

Experimental Evaluation of Microplasmin – An Alternative to Vital Dyes

Arnd Gandorfer

Vitreoretinal and Pathology Unit, Department of Ophthalmology, Ludwig-Maximilians-University, Munich, Germany

Abstract

Complete separation of the vitreous from the retina is a major goal of vitrectomy. Mechanical vitrectomy, however, is not able to meet this need because remnants of the vitreous cortex are left behind at the retinal surface, resulting in incomplete posterior vitreous detachment (PVD). As incomplete PVD and an attached vitreous cortex are associated with the progression of common retinal diseases including diabetic retinopathy and maculopathy, central retinal vein occlusion, and proliferative vitreoretinopathy, induction of complete PVD is a major issue both in vitreoretinal surgery and in medical retina. This chapter focuses on one of the most promising current concepts of pharmacologic vitreolysis, i.e. microplasmin-assisted vitrectomy. Microplasmin (Thrombogenics Ltd., Dublin, Ireland) is a recombinant molecule consisting of the catalytic domain of human plasmin. It shares the same catalytic properties like human plasmin, but it is much more stable compared to plasmin. It has been shown previously that both plasmin and microplasmin are capable of inducing PVD. Herein, we report on the preclinical work regarding plasmin and microplasmin which led to the clinical investigation of microplasmin.

The goal of enzymatic vitreolysis is to manipulate the vitreous collagen pharmacologically, both centrally achieving liquefaction (synchisis), as well as along the vitreoretinal interface to induce posterior vitreous detachment (PVD; syneresis), and to create a cleavage plane more safely and cleaner than can currently be achieved by mechanical means [1–4].

There are several reasons to pursue enzymatic-assisted vitreoretinal surgery. First, some retinal diseases that are currently managed in an operation room with mechanical manipulation of the vitreoretinal interface could be managed more safely by pharmacologic techniques or even in an office setting. Second, enzymatic-assisted

The author is the founder of the Microplasmin Study Group and has a financial interest in pharmacologic vitreolysis.

Table 1. Enzymes and effects of pharmacologic vitreolysis

Enzyme	Target	Effect
Chondroitinase	chondroitin sulfate	PVD in animal models
Hyaluronidase	hyaluronan	liquefaction
Dispase	type IV collagen	PVD, inner retinal damage
Plasmin/microplasmin	laminin and fibronectin MMP-2 activation	PVD and liquefaction

vitrectomy may achieve better anatomic and thus functional results by creating a cleaner cleavage plane between the vitreous and the retina than can be achieved currently by approaching the retina by mechanical means [1]. This is of particular importance in eyes with incomplete removal of the cortical vitreous from the retina, and in eyes with vitreoschisis, such as diabetic eyes [5]. Third, as incomplete PVD has been shown to be associated with both development of aggressive fibrovascular proliferation and macular edema, pharmacologic induction of complete PVD could prevent progression of diabetic retinopathy if given before advanced stages of diabetic eye disease [1, 6].

Several enzymes have been suggested as adjunctive therapy to vitreoretinal surgery or its replacement, including chondroitinase, hyaluronidase, dispase, and plasmin enzyme (table 1). In brief, chondroitinase, hyaluronidase, and dispase were of limited success due to insufficient vitreoretinal separation or digestion of inner retinal structures [7–13].

Plasmin, a nonspecific serine protease mediating the fibrinolytic process, also acts on a variety of glycoproteins including laminin and fibronectin, both of which are present at the vitreoretinal interface [14–16]. In 1993, PVD could be achieved in rabbit eyes by intravitreal injection of the enzyme followed by vitrectomy [17]. In 1999, Hikichi et al. [18] confirmed complete PVD after injection of 1 U plasmin and 0.5 ml SF_6 gas in the rabbit model, without evidence of retinal toxicity.

Plasmin is not available for clinical application, and alternative strategies have been pursued to administer the enzyme in vitreoretinal surgery. Tissue plasminogen activator was injected into the vitreous in an attempt to generate plasmin by intravitreal activation of endogenous plasminogen. In an animal model in rabbit eyes, complete PVD was observed in all eyes treated with 25 μg tissue plasminogen activator [19]. Breakdown of the blood-retinal barrier was necessary to allow plasminogen to enter the vitreous, and this was induced by cryocoagulation [19]. In two clinical pilot studies, 25 μg tissue plasminogen activator was injected into the vitreous of patients with proliferative diabetic retinopathy 15 min before vitrectomy [20, 21]. The results of both studies, however, were contradictory in terms of PVD induction and

Table 2. Grading system of cortical vitreous remnants at the vitreoretinal interface for scanning electron microscopy

Grading	Status of cortical vitreous
+++	no vitreoretinal separation
++	vitreoretinal separation, but continuous network of collagen fibrils on ILM
+	sparse collagen fibrils on ILM
–	bare ILM, no collagen fibrils

clinical benefit. Recently, Peyman's group [22] demonstrated PVD induction in rabbit eyes by an intravitreal administration of recombinant lysine-plasminogen and recombinant urokinase.

Autologous plasminogen purified from the patient's own plasma by affinity chromatography was converted to plasmin by streptokinase in vitro. 0.4 U of autologous plasmin enzyme was injected into the vitreous in patients with pediatric macular holes, diabetic retinopathy, and stage 3 idiopathic macular holes, followed by vitrectomy after 15 min [6, 23, 24]. In all eyes treated with autologous plasmin enzyme spontaneous or easy removal of the posterior hyaloid could be achieved including one eye that had vitreoschisis over areas of detached retina.

Development of Microplasmin-Assisted Vitrectomy

We investigated the effect of plasmin in porcine postmortem eyes and in human donor eyes. In porcine eyes, we observed a dose-dependent separation of the vitreous cortex from the internal limiting membrane (ILM) after intravitreal injection, without additional vitrectomy or gas injection [25]. In scanning electron microscopy, a bare ILM was achieved with 1 U of porcine plasmin 60 min after injection, and with 2 U of plasmin 30 and 60 min after injection. In control fellow eyes injected with balanced salt solution, the cortical vitreous remained attached to the retina [25]. We have developed a straightforward grading system that allows for easy and reliable quantification of cortical vitreous remnants at the ILM when scanning electron microscopy is performed (table 2) [25].

In human donor eyes, 2 U of human plasmin from pooled plasma achieved complete PVD 30 min after injection, whereas the vitreoretinal surface of the fellow eyes was covered by collagen fibrils [26]. In both studies, transmission electron microscopy revealed a clean and perfectly preserved ILM in plasmin-treated eyes, and no evidence of inner retinal damage was seen [25, 26]. Li et al. [27] confirmed these results,

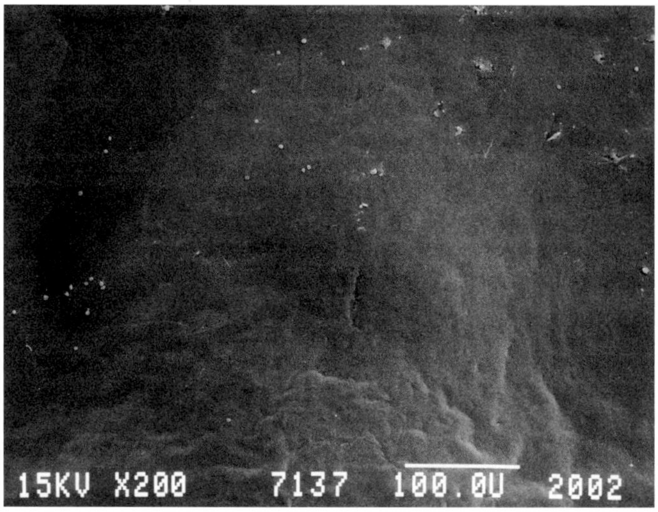

Fig. 1. Complete vitreoretinal separation following an intravitreal injection of microplasmin in a human donor eye.

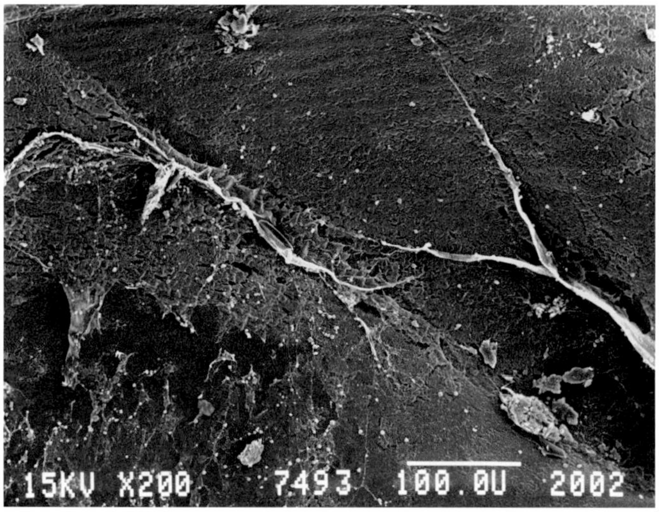

Fig. 2. Collagen remnants of the cortical vitreous at the vitreoretinal interface in a control eye.

and reported a reduced immunoreactivity of the vitreoretinal interface for laminin and fibronectin following plasmin application.

In an experimental setting simulating the application of plasmin as an adjunct to vitrectomy, we injected human donor eyes with 1 U of plasmin, followed by vitrectomy 30 min thereafter [28]. All plasmin-treated eyes showed complete PVD, whereas the control eyes which were vitrectomized conventionally had various amounts of the cortical vitreous still present at the vitreoretinal interface [28].

Recombinant microplasmin (Thrombogenics Ltd., Dublin, Ireland) is a truncated molecule containing the catalytic domain of human plasmin [29]. Microplasmin has the same catalytic properties as human plasmin, but is much more stable than the original molecule. It has been administered successfully into the vitreous of human [30] and porcine postmortem eyes (M. de Smet, Monte Carlo, 2004), and in rabbit and cat eyes in vivo [30, 31]. In all experimental settings, complete PVD was achieved in a dose-dependent fashion. No alteration of the inner retina was seen, and there was no change in antigenity of neurons and glial cells [30].

In 2001, we approached Thrombogenics Ltd., a drug development company which had manufactured recombinant microplasmin for clinical investigation in patients with stroke and peripheral artery occlusive disease. Given our preclinical work with human plasmin from pooled plasma, we tested microplasmin in human postmortem eyes in the same manner as we did before with human plasmin. There was a clear dose-response relationship of microplasmin comparable to that of human plasmin. Complete vitreoretinal separation was possible without affecting retinal morphology [30]. We went on testing the substance in the cat model in vivo. No alteration in retinal ultrastructure was seen, and there was no change in antigenity of neurons and glial cells [30]. This is important to know, as Müller cells are very sensitive to any form of ocular trauma and intraocular surgery. Further animal studies in different species followed. Formal toxicology testing was performed, and microplasmin entered the clinical phase. We designed the first clinical study investigating the effect of microplasmin in combination with vitrectomy (MIVI-I). This was done in collaboration with Marc de Smet and other members of the Microplasmin Study Group which was founded then. After having completed enrolment of patients for the MIVI-I trial, we went on designing a nonvitrectomy trial in patients with diabetic macular edema which is currently under way. The results of the MIVI-I study now serve as a basis for the FDA opening study starting in the USA.

Summary and Conclusion

Plasmin and microplasmin hold the promise of inducing complete PVD without causing morphologic alteration of the retina. Several independent studies confirmed a dose-dependent and complete vitreoretinal separation, associated with perfect preservation of the ultrastructure of the ILM and the retina [17, 18, 25, 26, 28, 30]. In addition, a dose-dependent liquefaction of the vitreous induced by microplasmin was demonstrated by dynamic light scattering in dissected porcine vitreous and in intact pig eyes (Ansari, Monte Carlo, 2004), making plasmin and microplasmin the most promising agents for pharmacologic vitreolysis at the moment. Clinical studies are now performed to assess the safety and efficacy of microplasmin when used as an adjunct to vitrectomy, or even as its replacement.

References

1 Trese M: Enzymatic-assisted vitrectomy. Eye 2002;16: 365–368.

2 Bhisitkul RB: Anticipation for enzymatic vitreolysis. Br J Ophthalmol 2001;85:1–2.

3 Sebag J: Pharmacologic vitreolysis. Retina 1998;18: 1–3.

4 Sebag J: Is pharmacologic vitreolysis brewing? Retina 2002;22:1–3.

5 Schwartz SD, Alexander R, Hiscott P, Gregor ZJ: Recognition of vitreoschisis in proliferative diabetic retinopathy. A useful landmark in vitrectomy for diabetic traction retinal detachment. Ophthalmology 1996;103:323–328.

6 Williams JG, Trese MT, Williams GA, Hartzer MK: Autologous plasmin enzyme in the surgical management of diabetic retinopathy. Ophthalmology 2001;108:1902–1905.

7 Hageman GS, Russell SR: Chondroitinase-mediated disinsertion of the primate vitreous body. Invest Ophthalmol Vis Sci 1994;35:1260.

8 Kuppermann BD, Thomas EL, de Smet MD, Grillone LR: Pooled efficacy results from two multinational randomized controlled clinical trials of a single intravitreous injection of highly purified ovine hyaluronidase (Vitrase) for the management of vitreous hemorrhage. Am J Ophthalmol 2005;140: 573–584.

9 Kuppermann BD, Thomas EL, de Smet MD, Grillone LR: Safety results of two phase III trials of an intravitreous injection of highly purified ovine hyaluronidase (Vitrase) for the management of vitreous hemorrhage. Am J Ophthalmol 2005;140: 585–597.

10 Hikichi T, Kado M, Yoshida A: Intravitreal injection of hyaluronidase cannot induce posterior vitreous detachment in the rabbit. Retina 2000;20:195–198.

11 Tezel TH, Del Priore LV, Kaplan HJ: Posterior vitreous detachment with dispase. Retina 1998;18:7–15.

12 Oliveira LB, Tatebayashi M, Mahmoud TH, Blackmon SM, Wong F, McCuen BW 2nd: Dispase facilitates posterior vitreous detachment during vitrectomy in young pigs. Retina 2001;21:324–331.

13 Jorge R, Oyamaguchi EK, Cardillo JA, Gobbi A, Laicine EM, Haddad A: Intravitreal injection of dispase causes retinal hemorrhages in rabbit and human eyes. Curr Eye Res 2003;26:107–112.

14 Kohno T, Sorgente N, Ishibashi T, Goodnight R, Ryan SJ: Immunofluorescent studies of fibronectin and laminin in the human eye. Invest Ophthalmol Vis Sci 1987;28:506–514.

15 Kohno T, Sorgente N, Goodnight R, Ryan SJ: Alterations in the distribution of fibronectin and laminin in the diabetic human eye. Invest Ophthalmol Vis Sci 1987;28:515–521.

16 Liotta LA, Goldfarb RH, Brundage R, Siegal GP, Terranova V, Garbisa S: Effect of plasminogen activator (urokinase), plasmin, and thrombin on glycoprotein and collagenous components of basement membrane. Cancer Res 1981;41:4629–4636.

17 Verstraeten TC, Chapman C, Hartzer M, Winkler BS, Trese MT, Williams GA: Pharmacologic induction of posterior vitreous detachment in the rabbit. Arch Ophthalmol 1993;111:849–854.

18 Hikichi T, Yanagiya N, Kado M, Akiba J, Yoshida A: Posterior vitreous detachment induced by injection of plasmin and sulfur hexafluoride in the rabbit vitreous. Retina 1999;19:55–58.

19 Hesse L, Nebeling B, Schroeder B, Heller G, Kroll P: Induction of posterior vitreous detachment in rabbits by intravitreal injection of tissue plasminogen activator following cryopexy. Exp Eye Res 2000;70:31–39.

20 Hesse L, Chofflet J, Kroll P: Tissue plasminogen activator as a biochemical adjuvant in vitrectomy for proliferative diabetic vitreoretinopathy. Ger J Ophthalmol 1995;4:323–327.

21 Le Mer Y, Korobelnik JF, Morel C, Ullern M, Berrod JP: TPA-assisted vitrectomy for proliferative diabetic retinopathy: results of a double-masked, multicenter trial. Retina 1999;19:378–382.

22 Men G, Peyman GA, Genaidy M, Kuo PC, Ghahramani F, Blake DA, Bezerra Y, Naaman G, Figueiredo E: The role of recombinant lysine-plasminogen and recombinant urokinase and sulfur hexafluoride combination in inducing posterior vitreous detachment. Retina 2004;24:199–209.

23 Margherio AR, Margherio RR, Hartzer M, Trese MT, Williams GA, Ferrone PJ: Plasmin enzyme-assisted vitrectomy in traumatic pediatric macular holes. Ophthalmology 1998;105:1617–1620.

24 Trese MT, Williams GA, Hartzer MK: A new approach to stage 3 macular holes. Ophthalmology 2000;107:1607–1611.

25 Gandorfer A, Putz E, Welge-Lussen U, Gruterich M, Ulbig M, Kampik A: Ultrastructure of the vitreoretinal interface following plasmin assisted vitrectomy. Br J Ophthalmol 2001;85:6–10.

26 Gandorfer A, Priglinger S, Schebitz K, Hoops J, Ulbig M, Ruckhofer J, Grabner G, Kampik A: Vitreoretinal morphology of plasmin-treated human eyes. Am J Ophthalmol 2002;133:156–159.

27 Li X, Shi X, Fan J: Posterior vitreous detachment with plasmin in the isolated human eye. Graefes Arch Clin Exp Ophthalmol 2002;240:56–62.

28 Gandorfer A, Ulbig M, Kampik A: Plasmin-assisted vitrectomy eliminates cortical vitreous remnants. Eye 2002;16:95–97.
29 Nagai N, Demarsin E, Van Hoef B, Wouters S, Cingolani D, Laroche Y, Collen D: Recombinant human microplasmin: production and potential therapeutic properties. J Thromb Haemost 2003;1: 307–313.
30 Gandorfer A, Rohleder M, Sethi C, Eckle D, Welge-Lussen U, Kampik A, Luthert P, Charteris D: Posterior vitreous detachment induced by microplasmin. Invest Ophthalmol Vis Sci 2004;45:641–647.
31 Sakuma T, Tanaka M, Mizota A, Inoue J, Pakola S: Safety of in vivo pharmacologic vitreolysis with recombinant microplasmin in rabbit eyes. Invest Ophthalmol Vis Sci 2005;46:3295–3299.

Arnd Gandorfer, MD
Vitreoretinal and Pathology Unit, Department of Ophthalmology
Ludwig-Maximilians-University, Mathildenstrasse 8
DE–80336 Munich (Germany)
Tel. +49 89 5160 3800, Fax +49 89 5160 4778, E-Mail arnd.gandorfer@med.uni-muenchen.de

Author Index

Altvater, A. 43

Bottós, J. 91

Chofflet, J. 35
Costa, E.F. 91

Enaida, H. 115

Farah, M.E. 29, 91
Furlani, B. 29, 91

Gandorfer, A. 69, 141, 153
Grisanti, S. 43

Haritoglou, C. 69, 141
Hörle, S. 35

Ishibashi, T. 115

Jackson, T.L. 126

Kaempf, S. 101
Kampik, A. 69

Lima, V. 91

Maia, M. 29, 91
Mennel, S. 35, 101
Meyer, C.H. XI, 1, 29, 35, 91, 101

Penha, F.M. 29, 91
Peters, S. 43

Rodrigues, E.B. 29, 91

Schmidt, J.C. 35, 101
Schüttauf, F. 141
Sebag, J. 5

Thaler, S. 141
Thumann, G. 101

Wollensak, G. 82

Subject Index

Alveolar theory, vitreous structure 5, 6
Autologous blood, intravitreous application 38, 39

Benzopurpine 4B, history of use 31
Biomicroscopy, vitreous imaging 13–15
Brilliant blue G (BBG)
  animal studies 111
  characteristics 33, 102, 103, 116, 118
  internal limiting membrane staining
      toxicity studies
    clinical studies
      pharmacological effects 121–123
      pilot study of membrane peeling 120, 121
    primate eye studies 119
    rat eyes
      intravitreous injection 118, 119
      subretinal injection 119
  osmolarity of solutions 116, 118
  retinal pigment epithelium effects
    transepithelial resistance studies 103, 104, 106, 107, 110, 111
    transmission electron microscopy studies 104, 108
Bromophenol blue (BPB)
  cell toxicity studies
    life-dead assay 145
    MTT assay 144, 145
  characteristics 33
  clinical staining of epiretinal membrane, vitreous, and lens capsule 147–150
  light-absorbing properties 144
  long-term toxicity studies
    histology 146, 147
    retinal ganglion cell count 147
  staining specificity evaluation 143, 144

Chicago blue (CB)
  cell toxicity studies
    life-dead assay 145
    MTT assay 144, 145
  clinical staining of epiretinal membrane and lens capsule 150, 151
  history of use 31
  light-absorbing properties 144
  long-term toxicity studies
    histology 146, 147
    retinal ganglion cell count 147
  staining specificity evaluation 143, 144
Chromovitrectomy
  historical perspective 32
  stain characteristics 32, 33
Collagen, vitreous composition 7, 8
Color contrast, dyes 134, 136

Dynamic light scattering (DLS), vitreous studies 23–25

E68 dye
  cell toxicity studies
    life-dead assay 145
    MTT assay 144, 145
  light-absorbing properties 144
  long-term toxicity studies
    histology 146, 147
    retinal ganglion cell count 147
  staining specificity evaluation 143, 144
Electroretinography (ERG)
  brilliant blue G studies 118
  indocyanine green toxicity studies 72, 73
  patent blue studies 110
Embryology
  internal limiting lamina 8, 9
  vitreous body 9–11

Enzyme-assisted vitrectomy, *see* Microplasmin-assisted vitrectomy
Epiretinal membrane (ERM)
bromophenol blue staining 147–150
Chicago blue staining 150, 151
holes 115
trypan blue staining 91, 93, 142
Evans blue, history of use 31

Fibrillar theory, vitreous structure 6
Fluorescein
characteristics 32
history of use 30, 31
preoperative fluorescein angiography and vitreous cortex visualization during vitreoretinal surgery 40
Fluorometholone, characteristics 33

Hyaluronan, vitreous composition 7, 8

India ink, history of use 30, 31
Indocyanine green (ICG)
characteristics 32, 44, 69
history of use 2, 44, 70
internal limiting membrane changes after staining
biomechanical effects
measurements 84
statistical evaluation 84
ultimate elongation 85, 86
ultimate force 85, 86
illumination and spectroscopy 84, 85, 87
overview 82, 83
specimen preparation 83
staining protocol 83
thickness measurements 84, 85
treatment groups 83
osmolarity of solutions 116
photooxidative damage 87
retinal toxicity
adverse events in internal limiting membrane peeling 77, 78
animal studies of intravitreal injection
rabbit 73
rat 72, 73
ex vivo models 74–76
in vitro studies 71, 72
overview 45, 59
postmortem findings 70, 71
subretinal injection in rabbit 75
vitrectomy and internal limiting membrane staining in cat 74
safety parameters in vitreoretinal surgery
clinical experience 46–51
dye persistence effects 51–54
exposure time 50, 51
osmolarity effects 58–60
phototoxicity and illumination time 54–57, 60
preclinical data interpretation 46
protocol establishment 45
solution preparation 69
structure 44, 70
Internal limiting lamina (ILL)
embryology 8, 9
neovascularization 9
Internal limiting membrane (ILM)
anatomy 82
brilliant blue G staining 111, 116, 118
cross-linking 89
function 115
peeling in macular surgery 37, 77, 120, 121, 141
triamcinolone in visualization 40
trypan blue staining 91, 93, 94
Interphotoreceptor matrix (IPM), vital staining 131, 132

Kiton fast green V, history of use 30
Kroll, Peter (vitreoretinal surgeon) 1–3

Lamellar theory, vitreous structure 6
Lens capsule
bromophenol blue staining 147–150
Chicago blue staining 150, 151
Light green SF yellowish (LG SF)
cell toxicity studies
life-dead assay 145
MTT assay 144, 145
light-absorbing properties 144
long-term toxicity studies
histology 146, 147
retinal ganglion cell count 147
staining specificity evaluation 143, 144

Methylene blue, history of use 31
Microplasmin-assisted vitrectomy
development 155–157
prospects 157
rationale 153–155
MTT assay, dye toxicity evaluation 144, 145

Nuclear magnetic resonance (NMR), vitreous studies 22

Ophthalmoscopy
conventional imaging 12, 13
scanning laser ophthalmoscopy 15, 16
Optical coherence tomography (OCT)
combined optical coherence tomography-scanning laser ophthalmoscopy 18–22
vitreous imaging 17

Patent blue (PB)
animal studies 109, 110
characteristics 33, 102
history of use 33
retinal pigment epithelium effects
transepithelial resistance studies 103–105, 108, 109
transmission electron microscopy studies 104, 108
Plasmin, *see* Microplasmin-assisted vitrectomy
Posterior vitreous detachment (PVD)
imaging 13, 16, 20, 21
induction of complete detachment, *see* Microplasmin-assisted vitrectomy
Proliferative diabetic vitreoretinopathy, histology 11, 12
Purinergic receptor, brilliant blue G antagonism 121–123
PVD, *see* Posterior vitreous detachment

Radial sector theory, vitreous structure 6
Raman spectroscopy, vitreous studies 22, 23
Retina
brilliant blue G effects
transepithelial resistance studies 103, 104, 106, 107, 110, 111
transmission electron microscopy studies 104, 108
indocyanine green toxicity, *see* Indocyanine green
patent blue effects
transepithelial resistance studies 103–105, 108, 109
transmission electron microscopy studies 104, 108
retinal pigment epithelium structure 102
tearing point 88
trypan blue
staining of breaks 94
toxicity, *see* Trypan blue
Retinal detachment surgery
outcomes 126, 127
vital staining
chromophore stains 128, 129
color contrast 134, 136
fluorophore stains 129, 130
historical perspective 127, 128
targets
dead cells 132, 133
interphotoreceptor matrix 131, 132
intracellular constituents 133, 134
retinal pigment epithelium 131
trypan blue 136–139
Rhodamine 6G
cell toxicity studies
life-dead assay 145
MTT assay 144, 145
light-absorbing properties 144
long-term toxicity studies
histology 146, 147
retinal ganglion cell count 147
staining specificity evaluation 143, 144
Rhodulirein blue 3G
cell toxicity studies
life-dead assay 145
MTT assay 144, 145
light-absorbing properties 144
long-term toxicity studies
histology 146, 147
retinal ganglion cell count 147
staining specificity evaluation 143, 144

Scanning laser ophthalmoscopy (SLO)
combined optical coherence tomography-scanning laser ophthalmoscopy 18–22
vitreous imaging 15, 16

Transepithelial resistance (TER)
brilliant blue G effects on retinal pigment epithelium 103, 104, 106, 107, 110, 111
patent blue effects on retinal pigment epithelium 103–105, 108, 109
Transmission electron microscopy (TEM)
brilliant blue G effects on retinal pigment epithelium 104, 108
patent blue effects on retinal pigment epithelium 104, 108
Triamcinolone
characteristics 33
history of use 39

Triamcinolone (continued)
vitreous cortex visualization during
vitreoretinal surgery 39, 40
Trypan blue (TB)
applications 92, 93
characteristics 32, 92
chromovitrectomy use 93–95
dilution in glucose 98
epiretinal membrane staining 91, 93, 142
history of use 31, 33, 91
osmolarity of solutions 116
retinal detachment surgery 136–139
retinal toxicity
animal studies 96, 97
in vitro studies 95, 96
staining specificity 91, 93, 94
structure 92
Trypan red, history of use 31
Tyndall effect, biomicroscopy 13–15

Ultrasonography, vitreous imaging 16

Vitreous
bromophenol blue staining 147–150
collagen 7, 8
dynamic light scattering 23–25
embryology
internal limiting lamina 8, 9
vitreous body 9–11
function 142
history of study 5–7
hyaluronan 7, 8
imaging
biomicroscopy 13–15
combined optical coherence
tomography-scanning laser
ophthalmoscopy 18–22
in vitro 11, 12
nuclear magnetic resonance 22
ophthalmoscopy 12, 13
optical coherence tomography 17
Raman spectroscopy 22, 23
scanning laser ophthalmoscopy 15, 16
ultrasonography 16
staining rationale 142
structure 5, 6
supramolecular organization 8
trypan blue staining 94
Vitreous cortex
visualization during vitreoretinal surgery
autologous blood intravitreous
application 38, 39
preoperative fluorescein angiography
40
triamcinolone acetonide 39, 40
vitrectomy indications 35, 36, 41